Getting Ready for™ My Brain Surgery

A Brain Surgery Book for Kids - Preparation and Recovery

This book belongs to:

____

Written by Dr. Fei Zheng-Ward Illustrated by Moch. Fajar Shobaru

Identifiers: ISBN 979-8-89318-182-1 (eBook)
ISBN 979-8-89318-183-8 (paperback)
ISBN 979-8-89318-184-5 (hardcover)

Your brain is amazing!

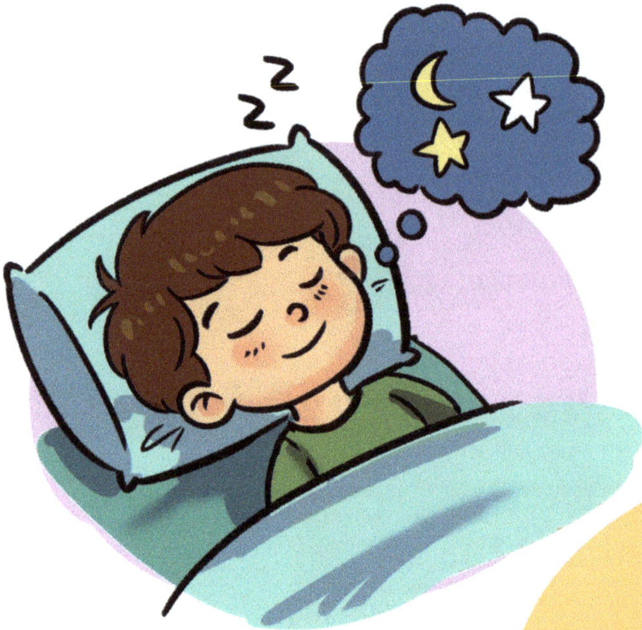

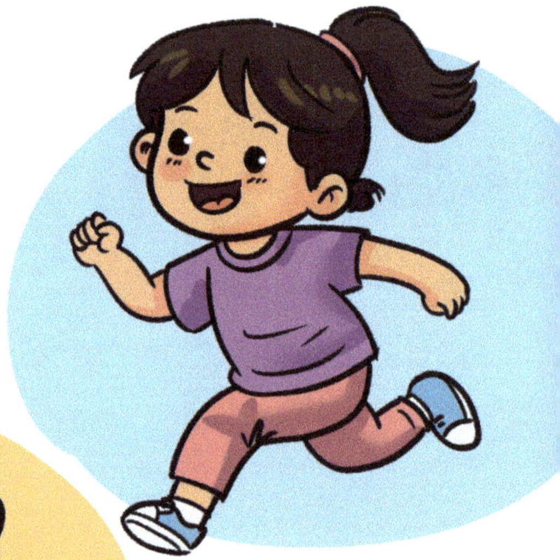

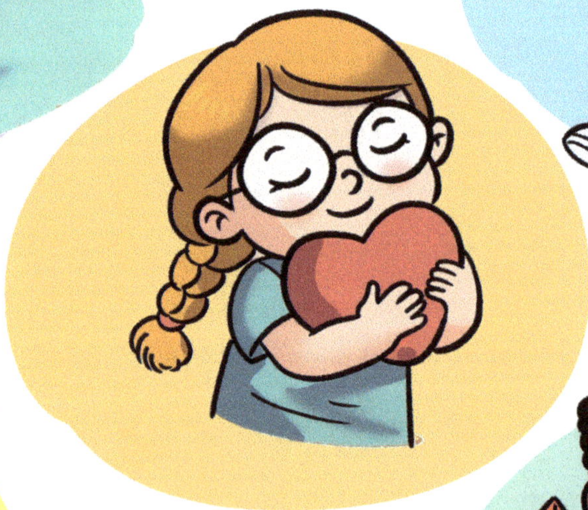

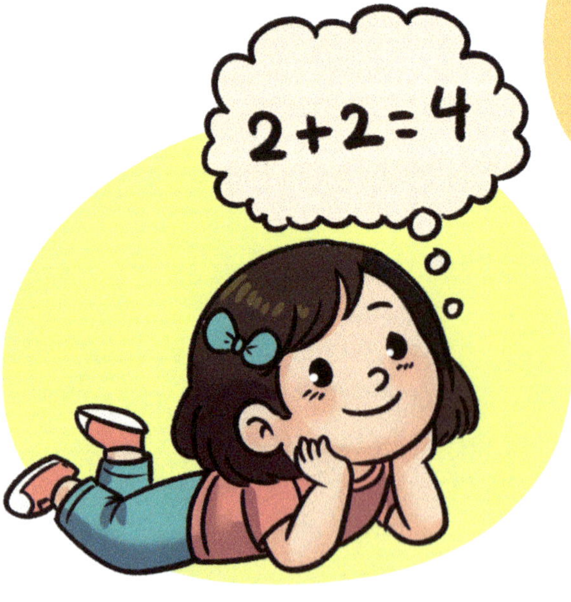

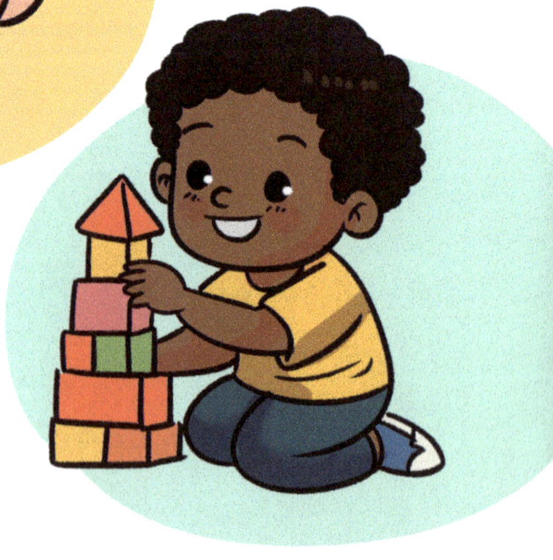

It helps you think, move, feel, talk, play, and dream.

Just like any other part of the body, sometimes the brain needs a little help.

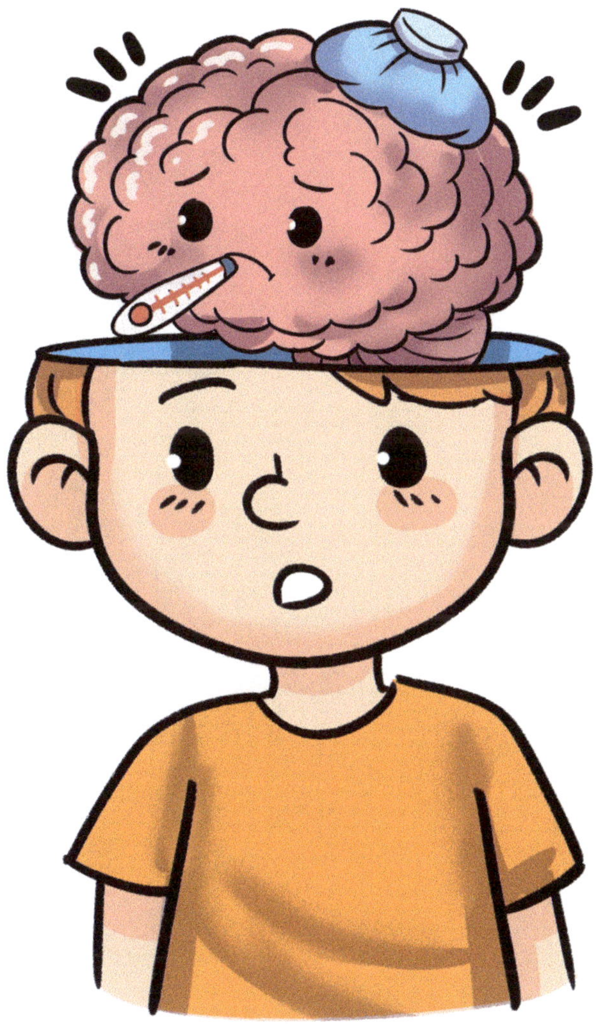

Sometimes, when the brain isn't feeling its best, some kids may experience:

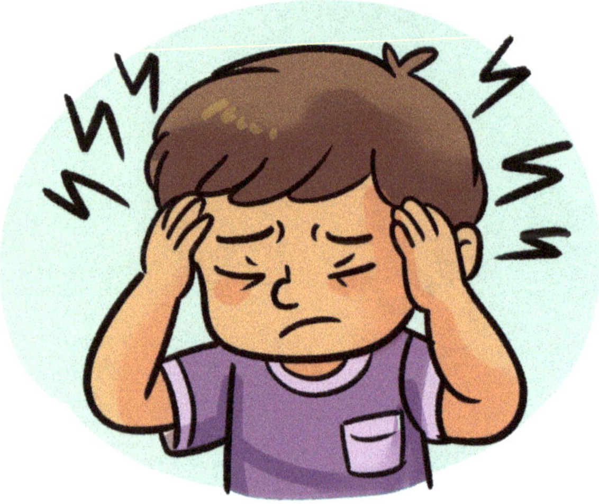

☐ Headaches

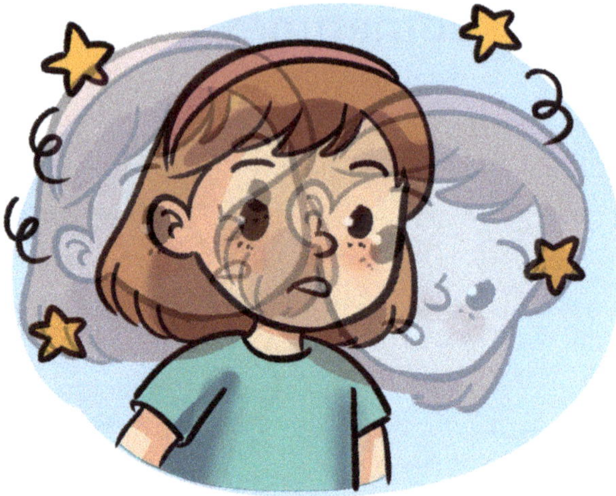

☐ Trouble seeing

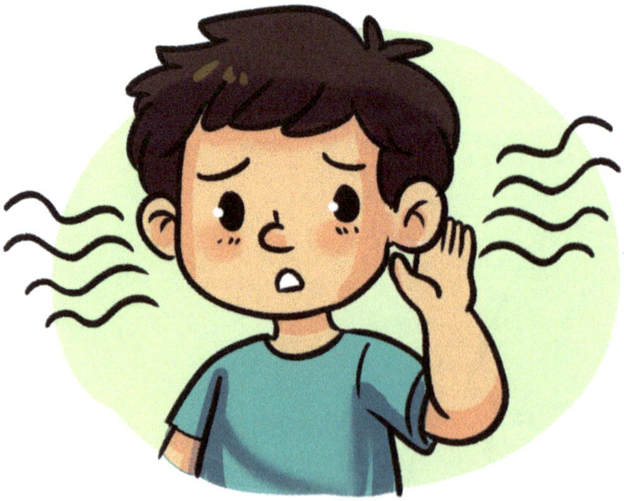

☐ Feeling, smelling, or hearing something unusal

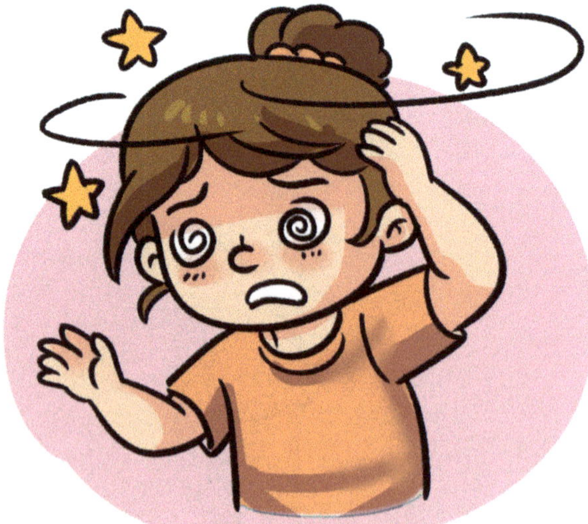

☐ Feeling dizzy

☐ Feeling tired

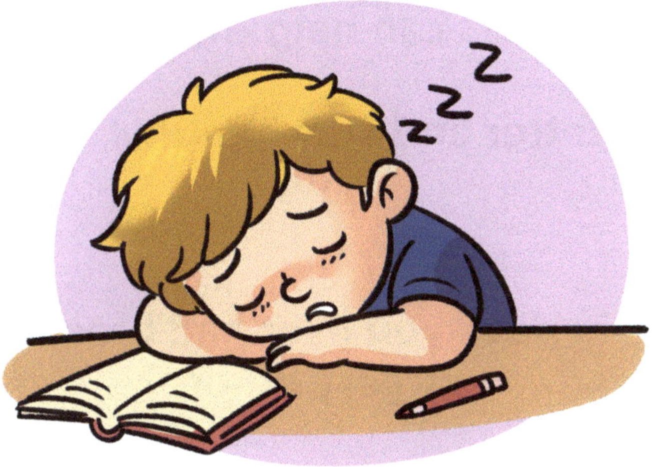

☐ Feeling nauseous or sick to your tummy

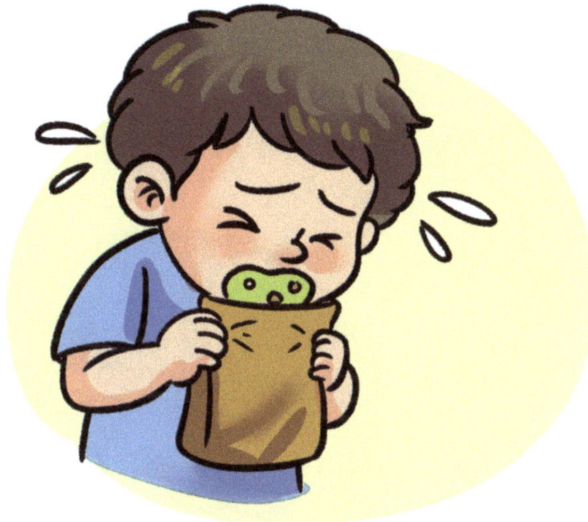

☐ Not feeling like your normal self

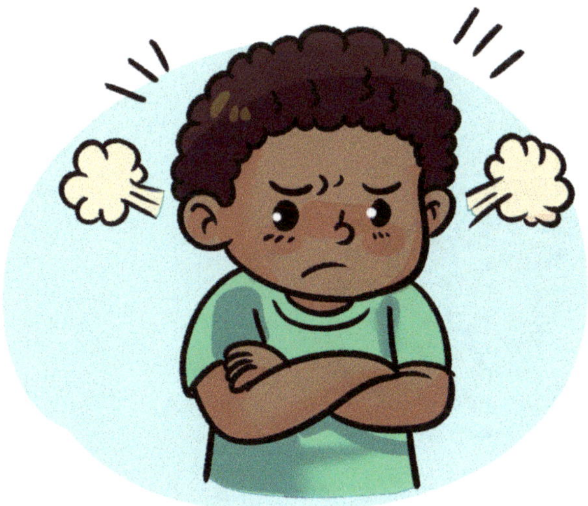

☐ A sleepy or tingly arm or leg

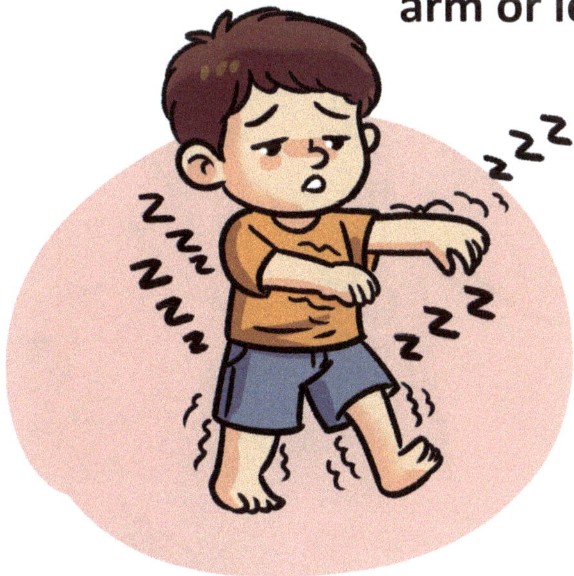

What have you experienced?
You can mark them above.

Brain surgery is a special way doctors can help the brain.

They help your brain work better and stay healthy.

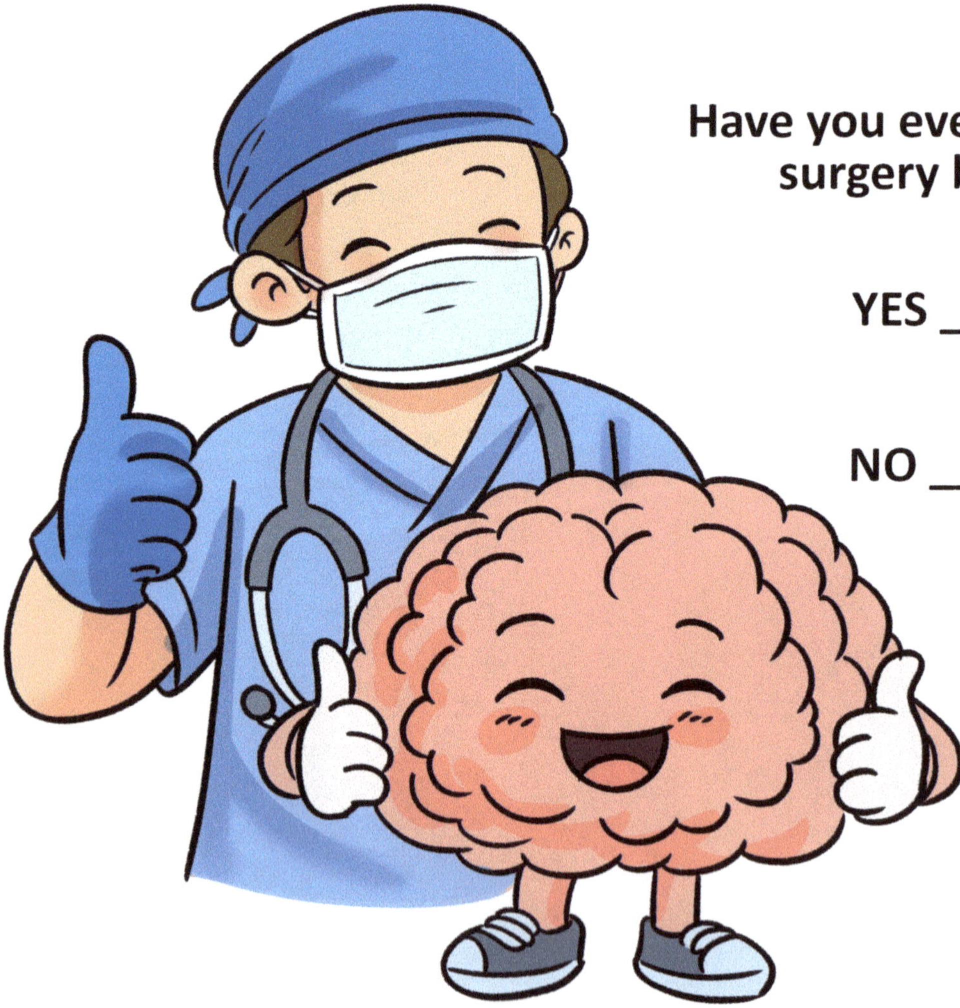

Have you ever had brain surgery before?

YES ____

NO ____

Every brain is different.

Here are some reasons a brain may need surgery.

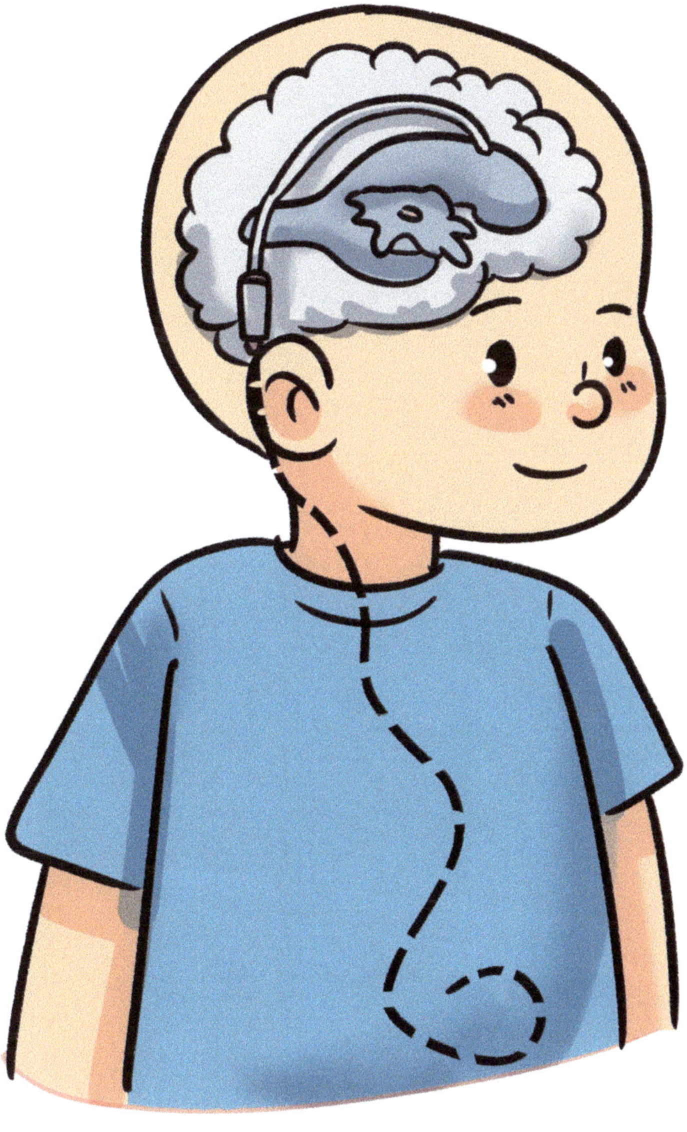

The brain has a special liquid that helps protect it, and sometimes there is too much of it.

Doctors may place a tiny tube called a shunt to help the liquid flow the right way.

Sometimes a small spot grows in the brain where it shouldn't. Doctors can remove it to give the brain more space and help it work better.

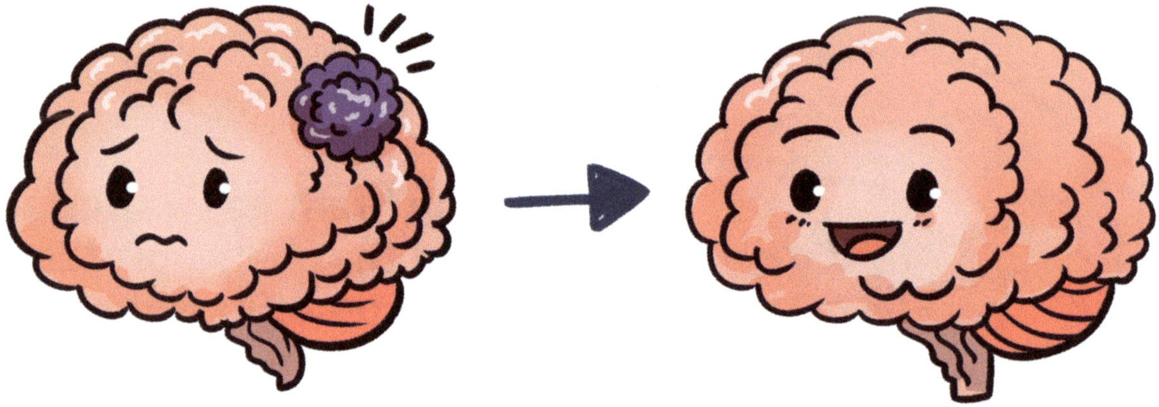

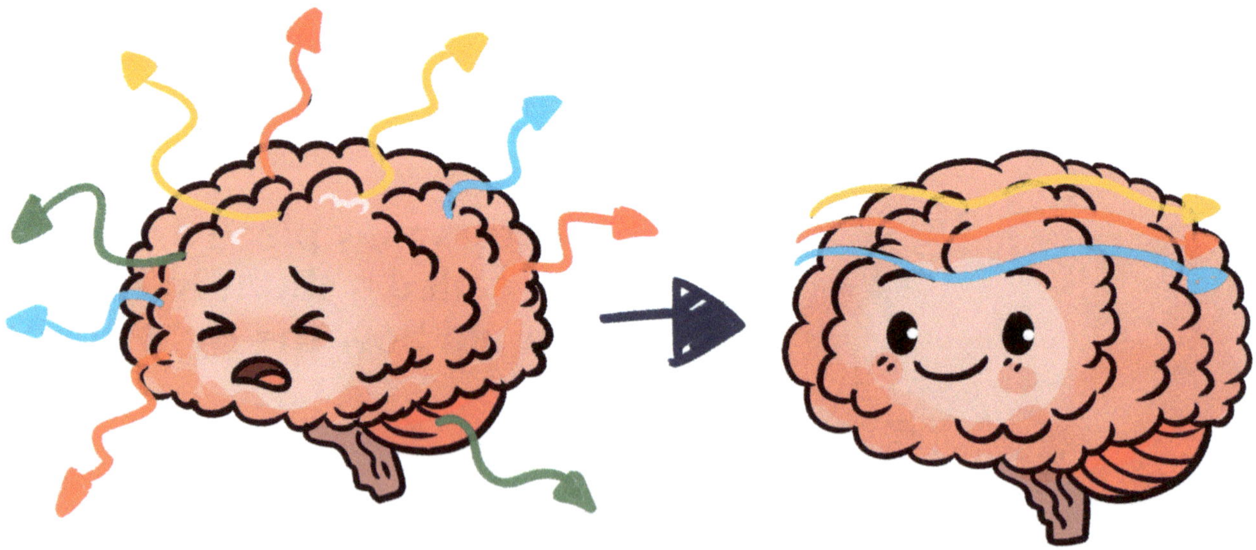

Some brains send mixed-up tiny messages all at once.
That can cause seizures.
Doctors can help the brain send calmer,
more organized messages.

Sometimes the brain feels a little crowded.
Doctors can help make more room so everything fits and works better.

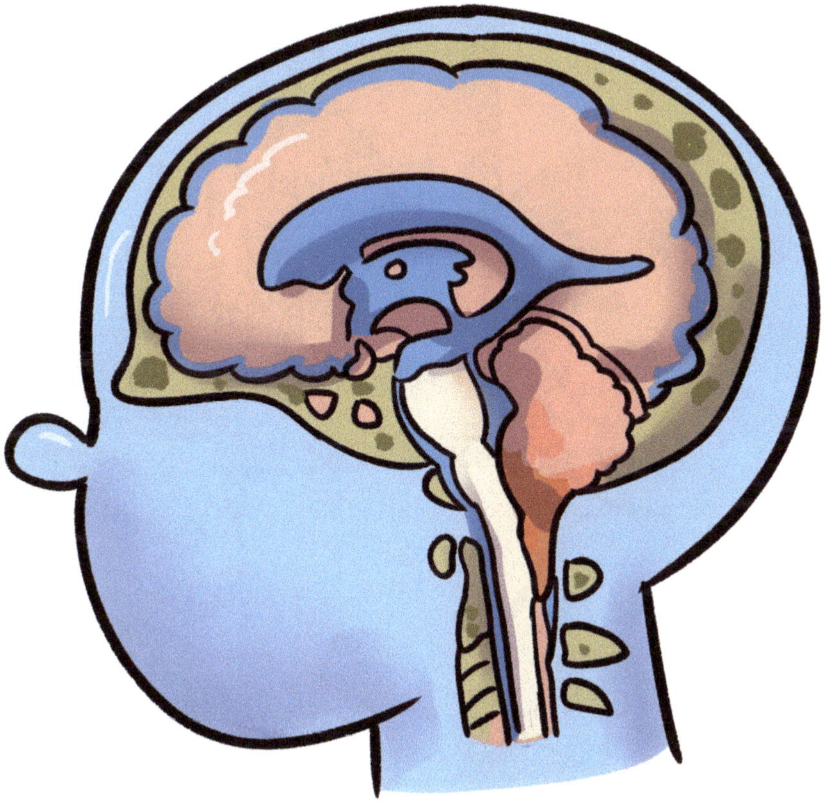

Many kids feel much better after their surgery.

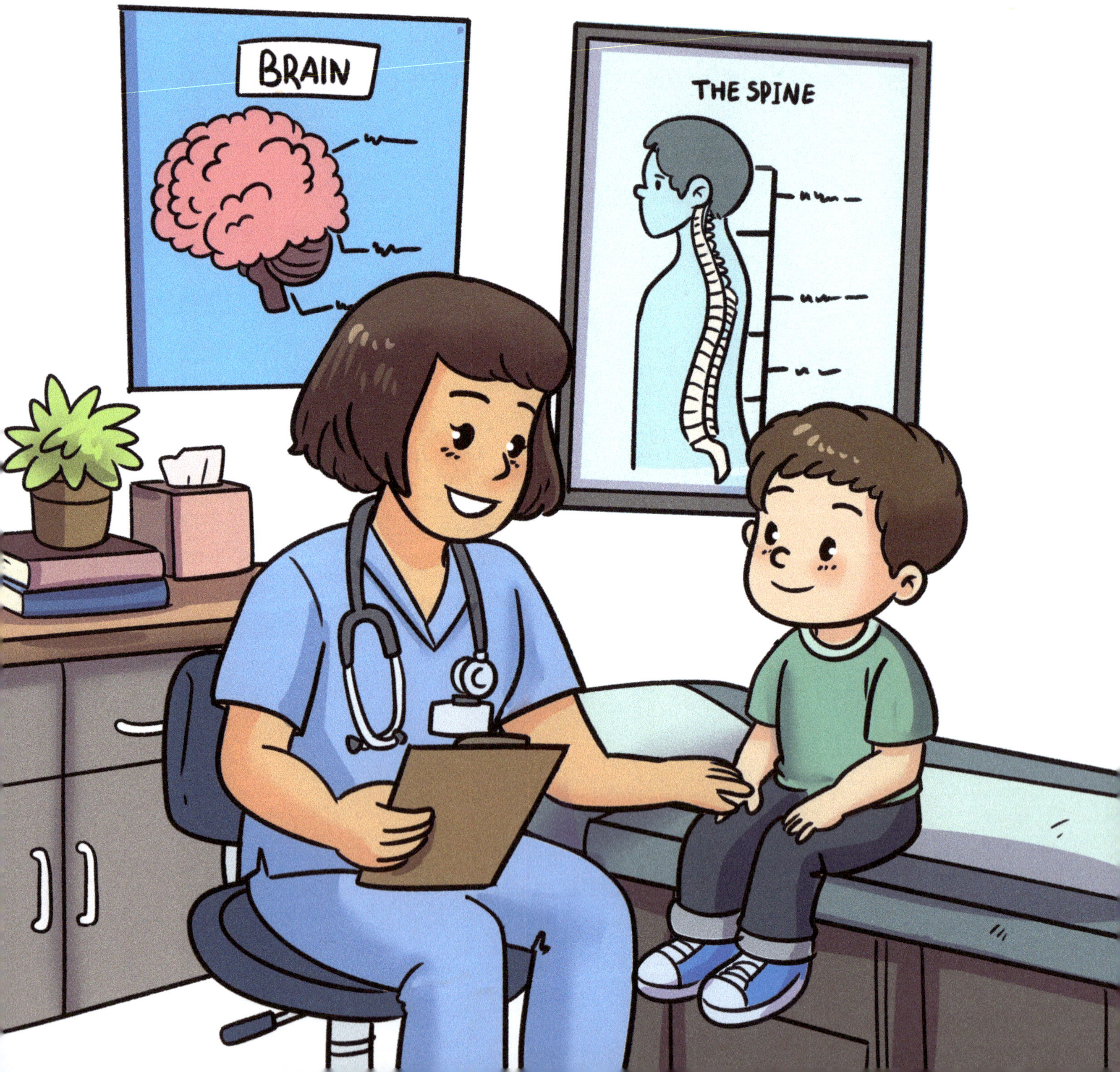
BRAIN
THE SPINE

Before your surgery, you may visit your surgery and anesthesia doctors to help you get ready.

They will explain how they will help you and how your body will heal afterward.

It's always okay to ask questions.

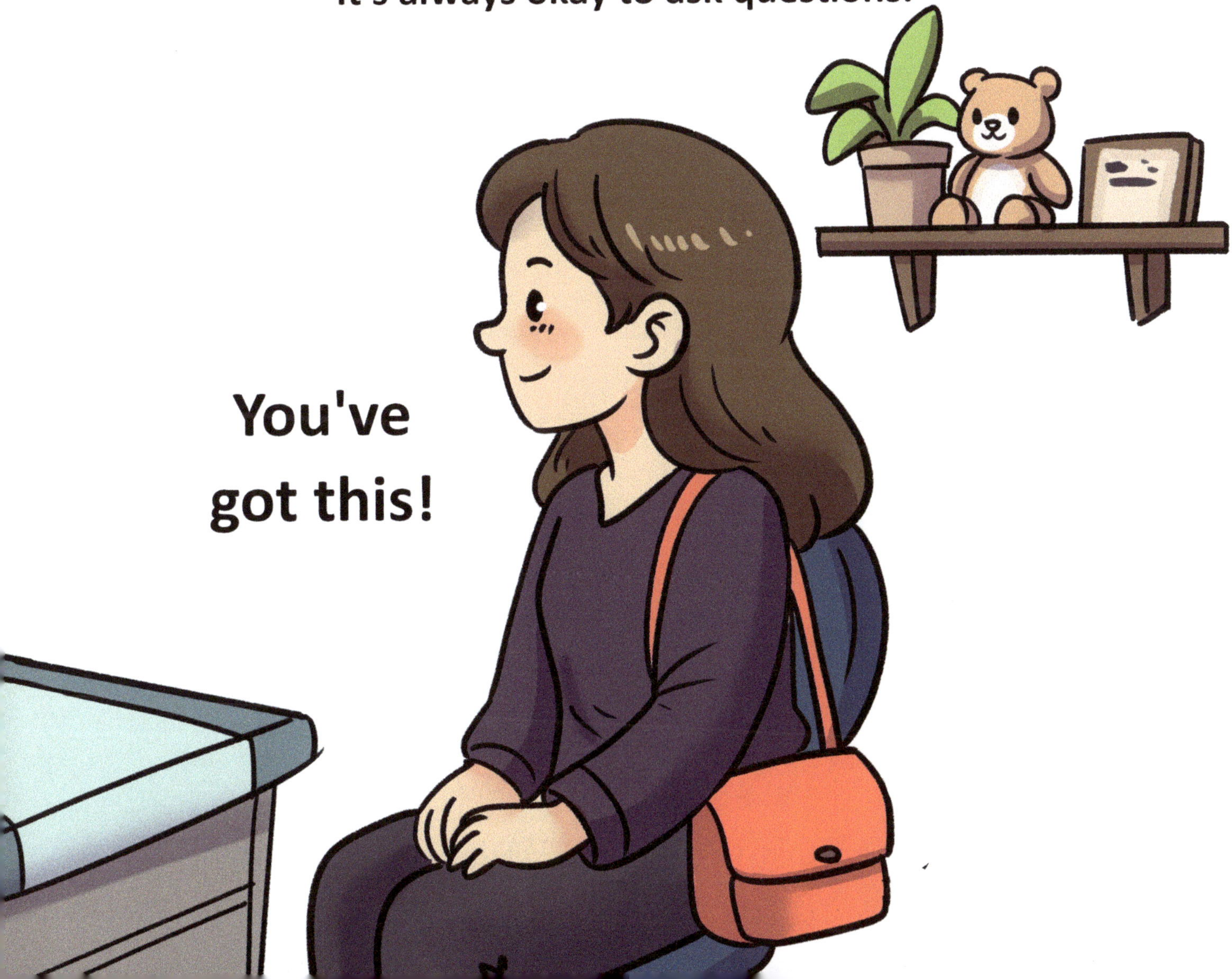

Before surgery, you may have:

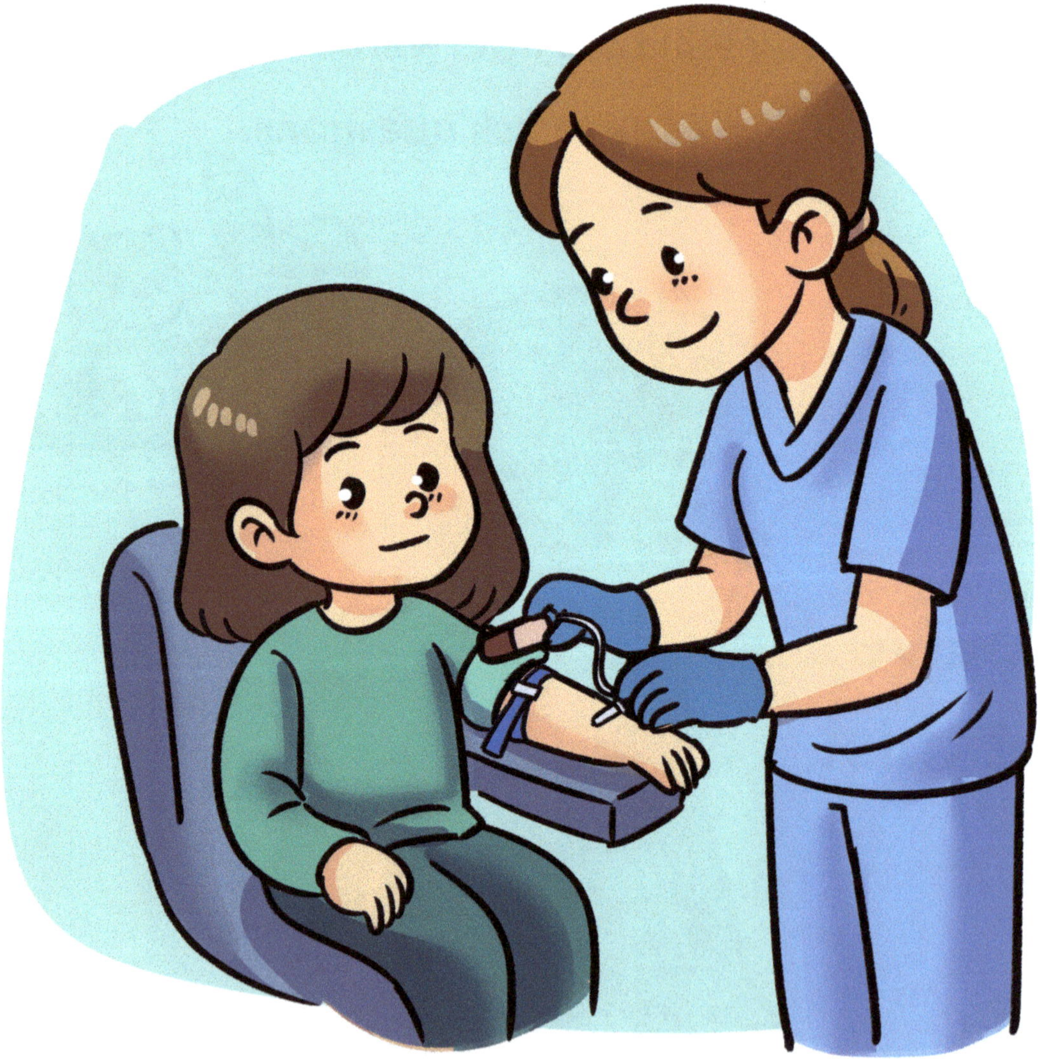

• A blood test to see how your body is doing

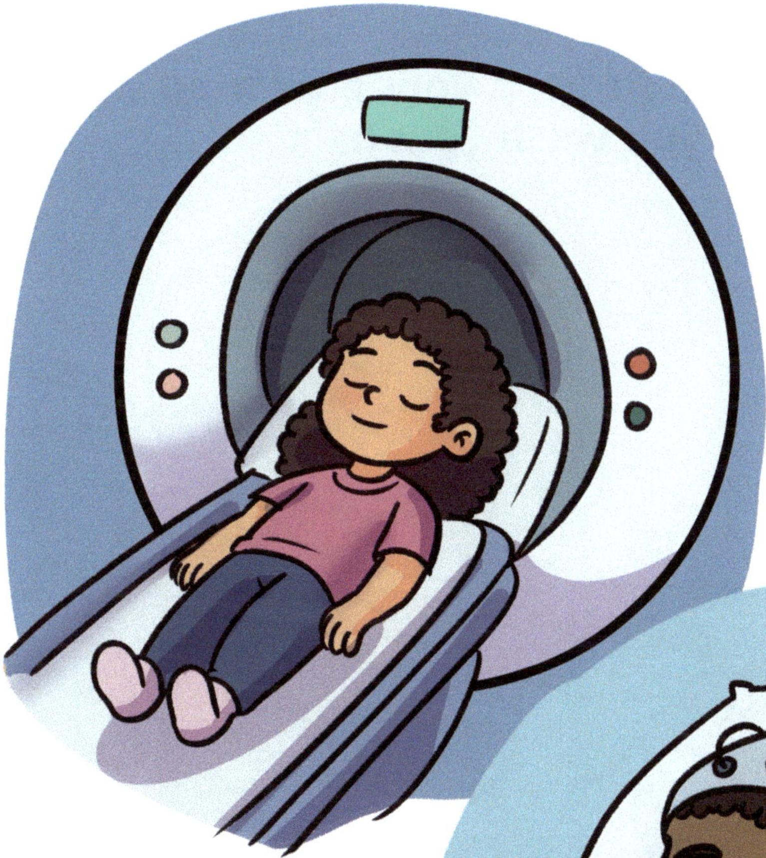

• Pictures of your brain called scans

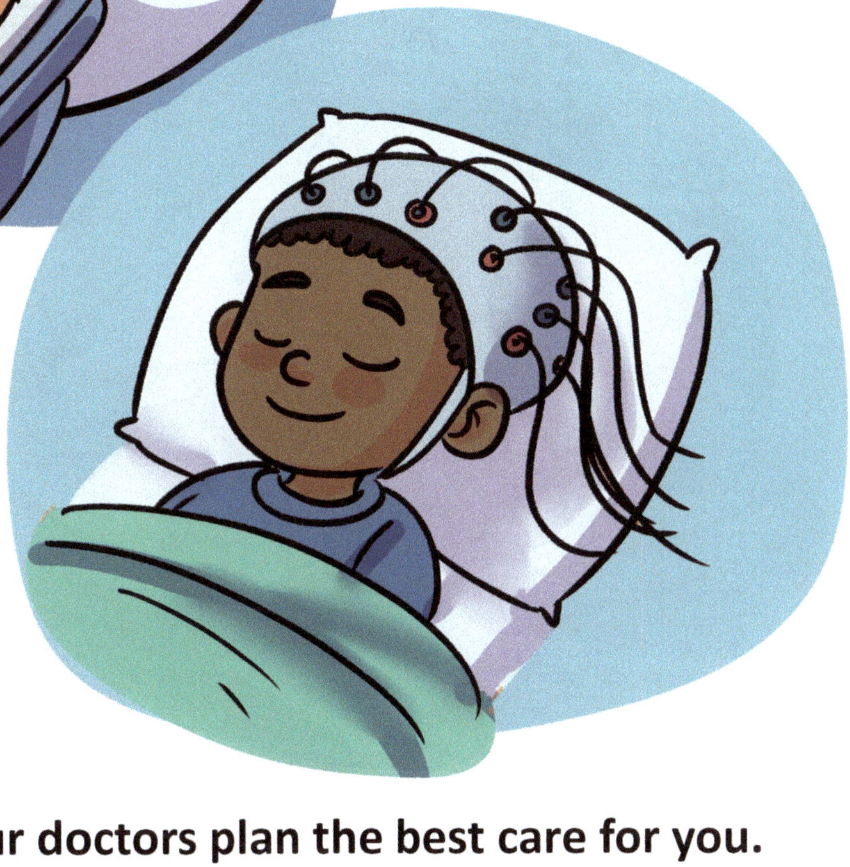

• A test that looks at brain signals, called an EEG

These tests help your doctors plan the best care for you.

The night before surgery, your grown-up will help you wash your hair.

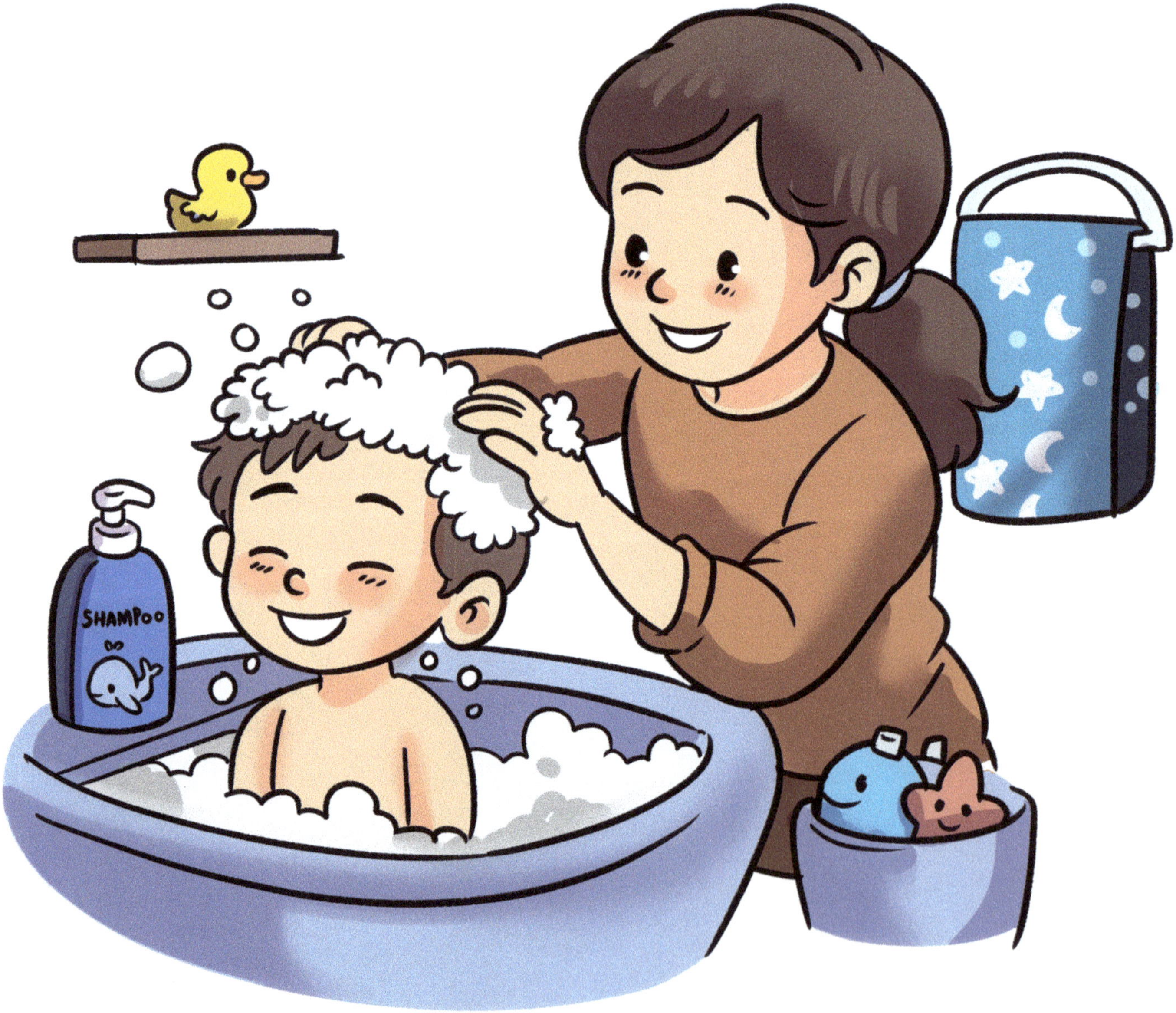

Your hair will be clean and free of oils or lotions.

You may also use special soap or wipes for your body.

This helps keep you safe and healthy.

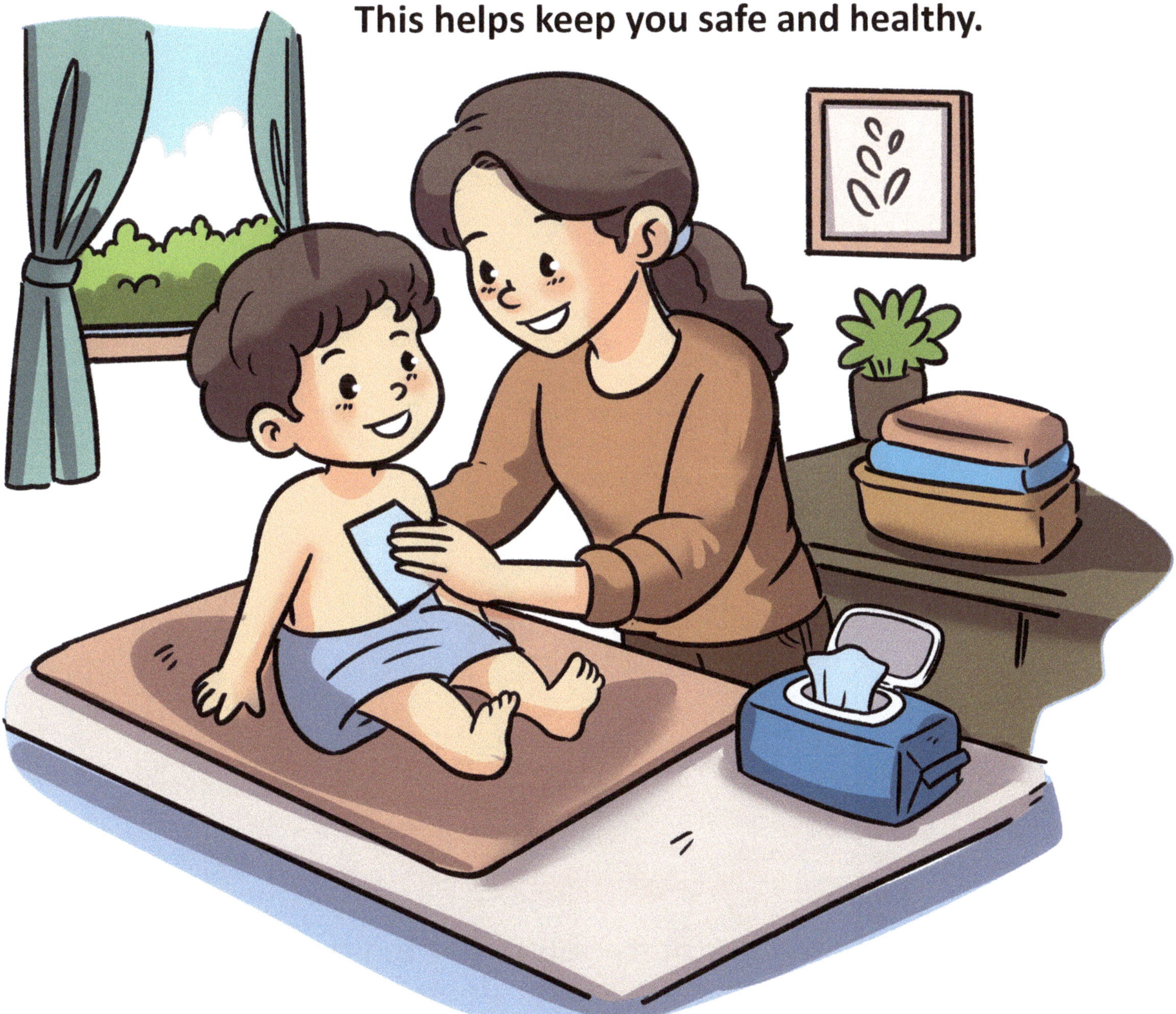

On the morning of surgery, you will skip breakfast.

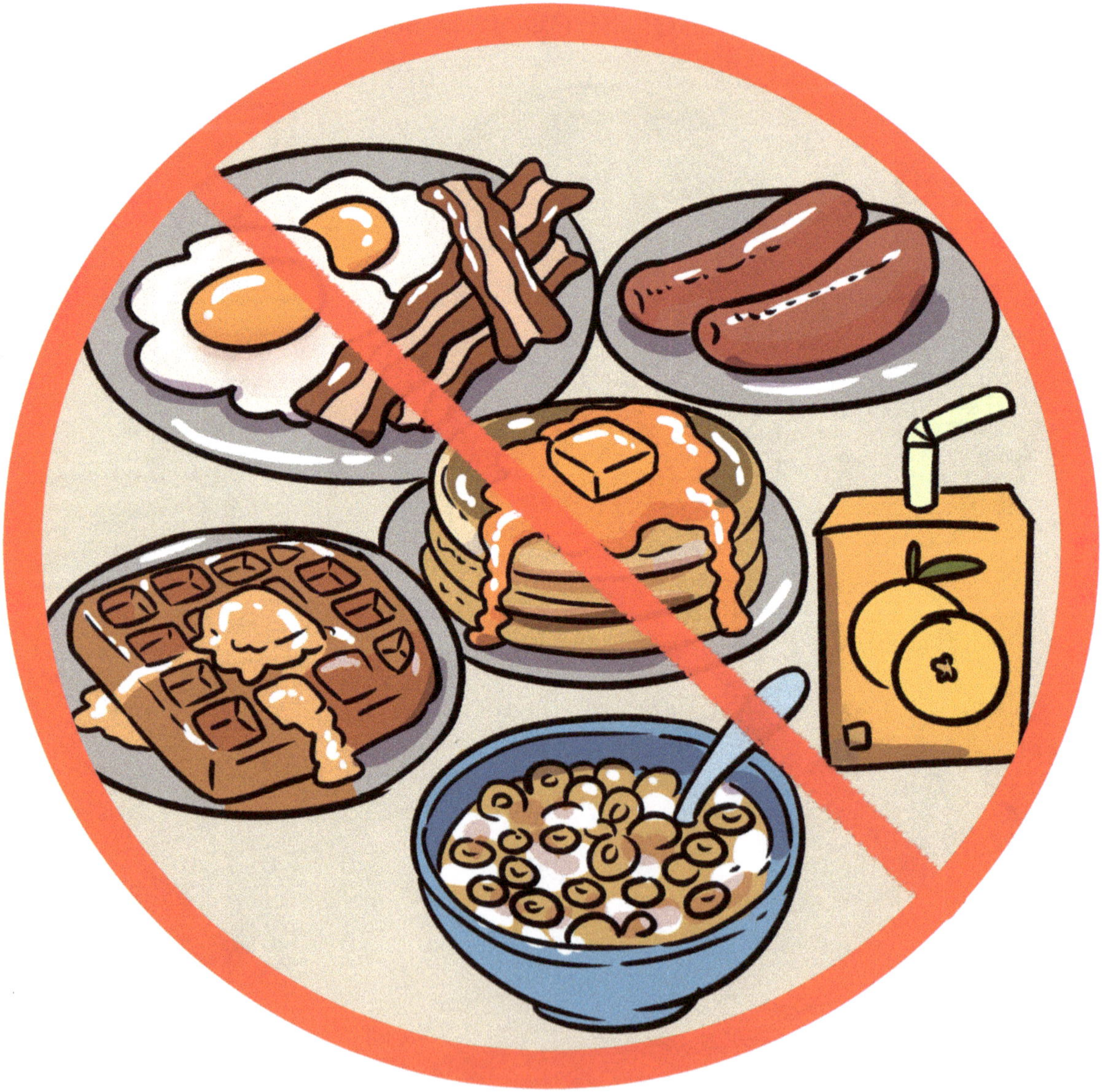

This tells your body you're getting ready and helps it stay safe while you sleep during surgery.

Your doctors and nurses will come say hello.

They are there just for you,
keeping you safe and comfortable.

You may get a special medicine to help you feel more calm.

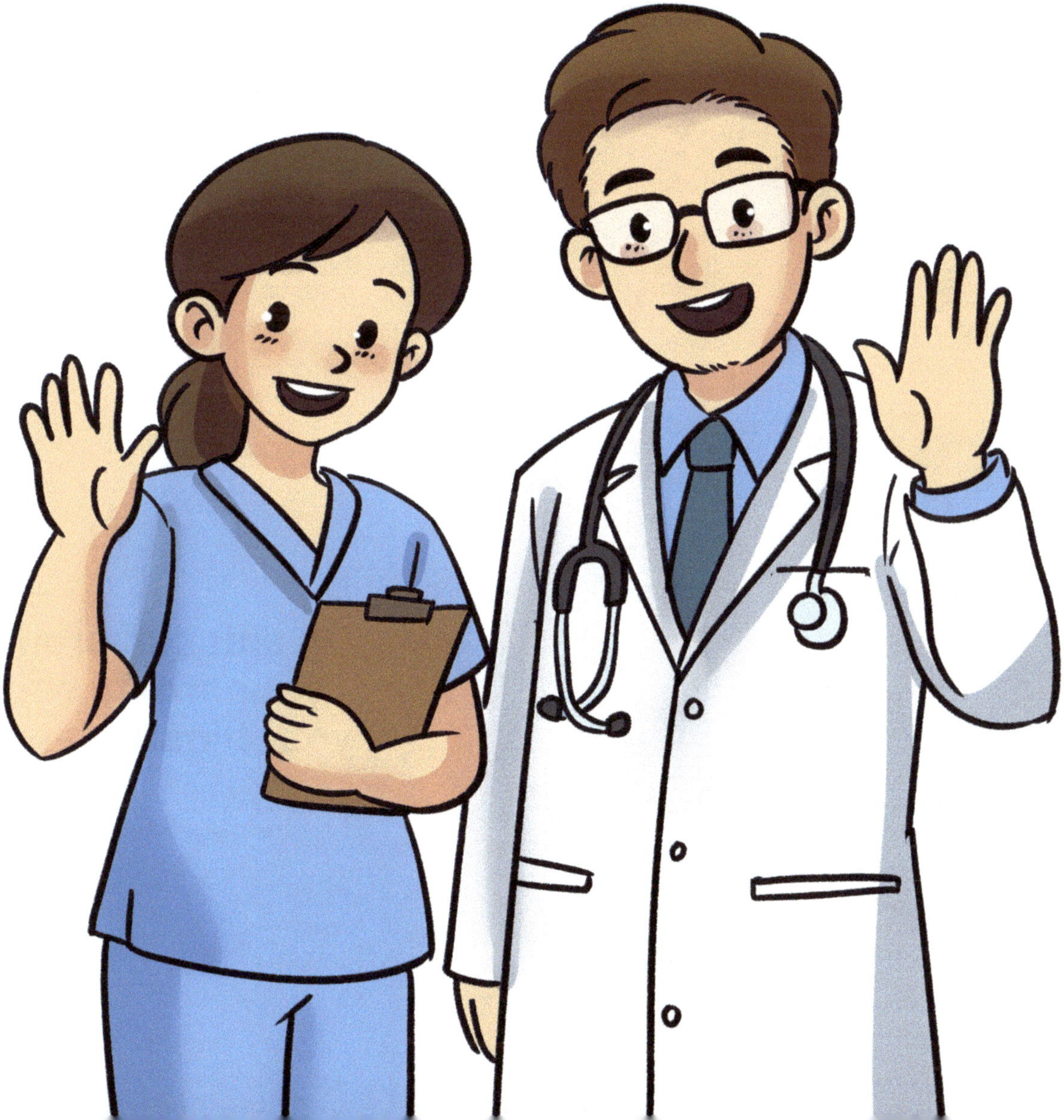

You may see some helpful medical tools:

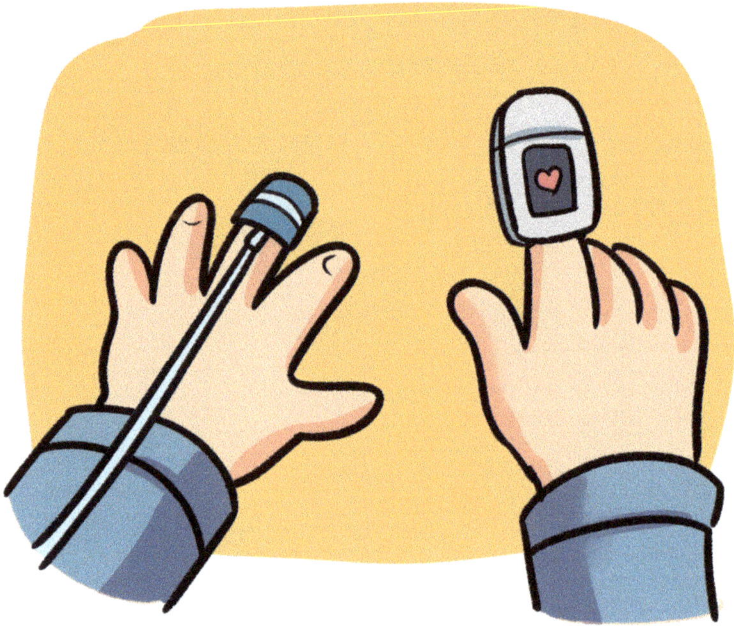

A clip or sticker on your finger to check oxygen (called a pulse oximeter, or pulse ox).

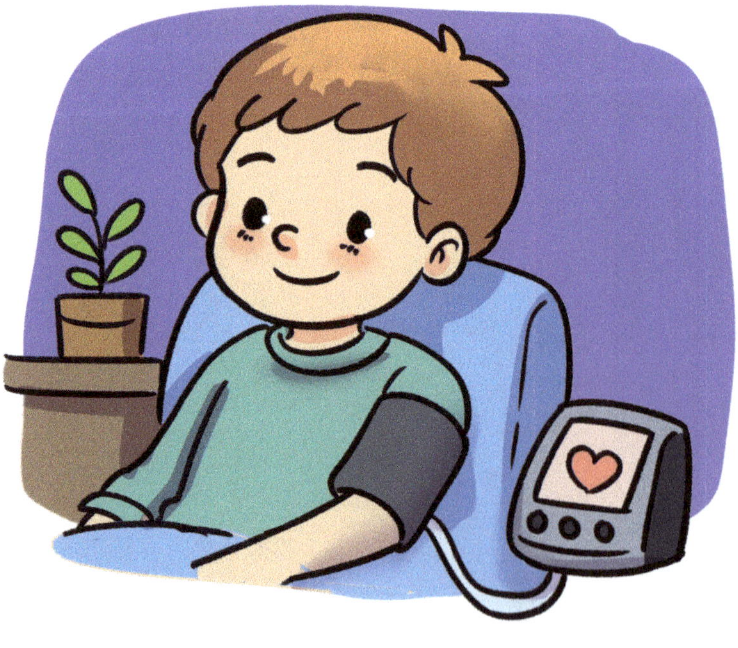

A soft cuff around your arm to check your blood pressure.

You're so brave!

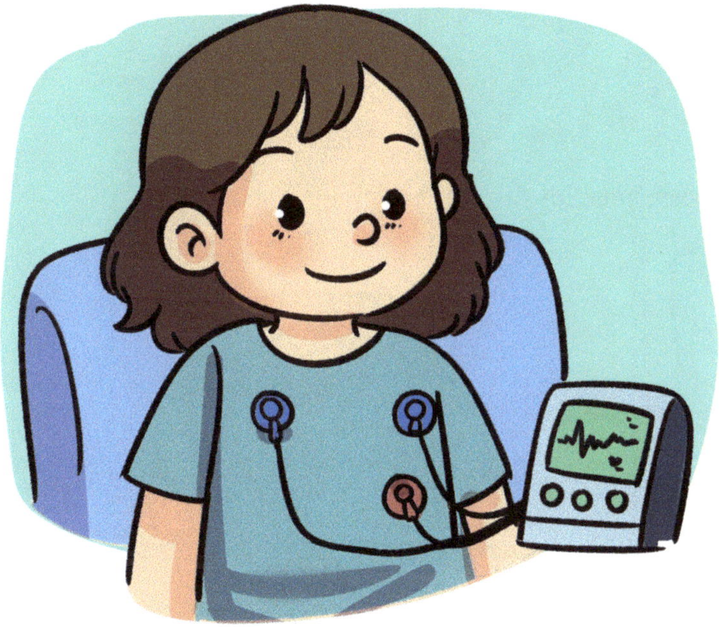

A few heart monitor stickers on your chest to check your heart.

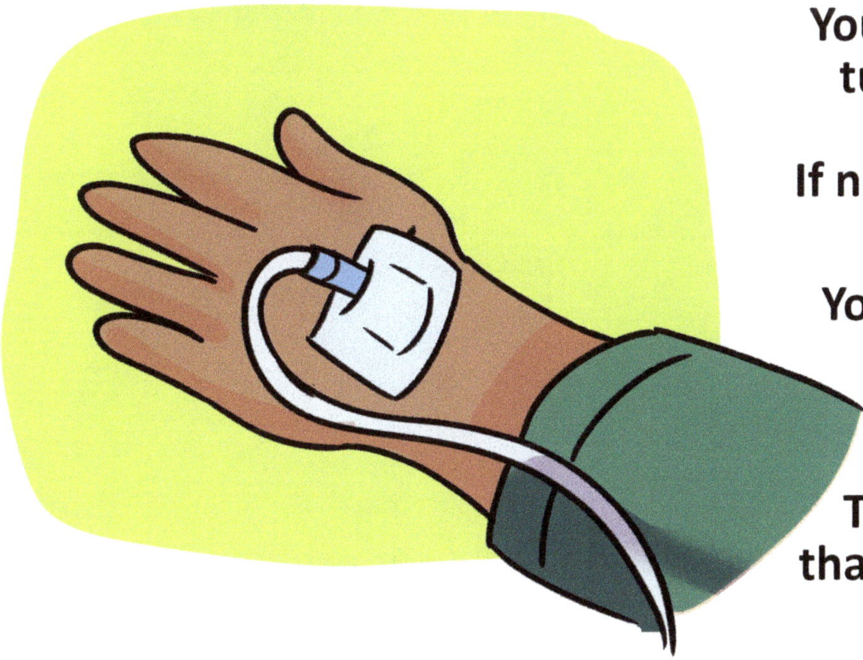

You may already have a tiny tube in your hand or arm called an IV.
If not, it can be placed before or after you’re asleep.

Your care team will choose the safest way for you.

The IV is like a tiny straw that gives your body fluids (a drink) and medicine.

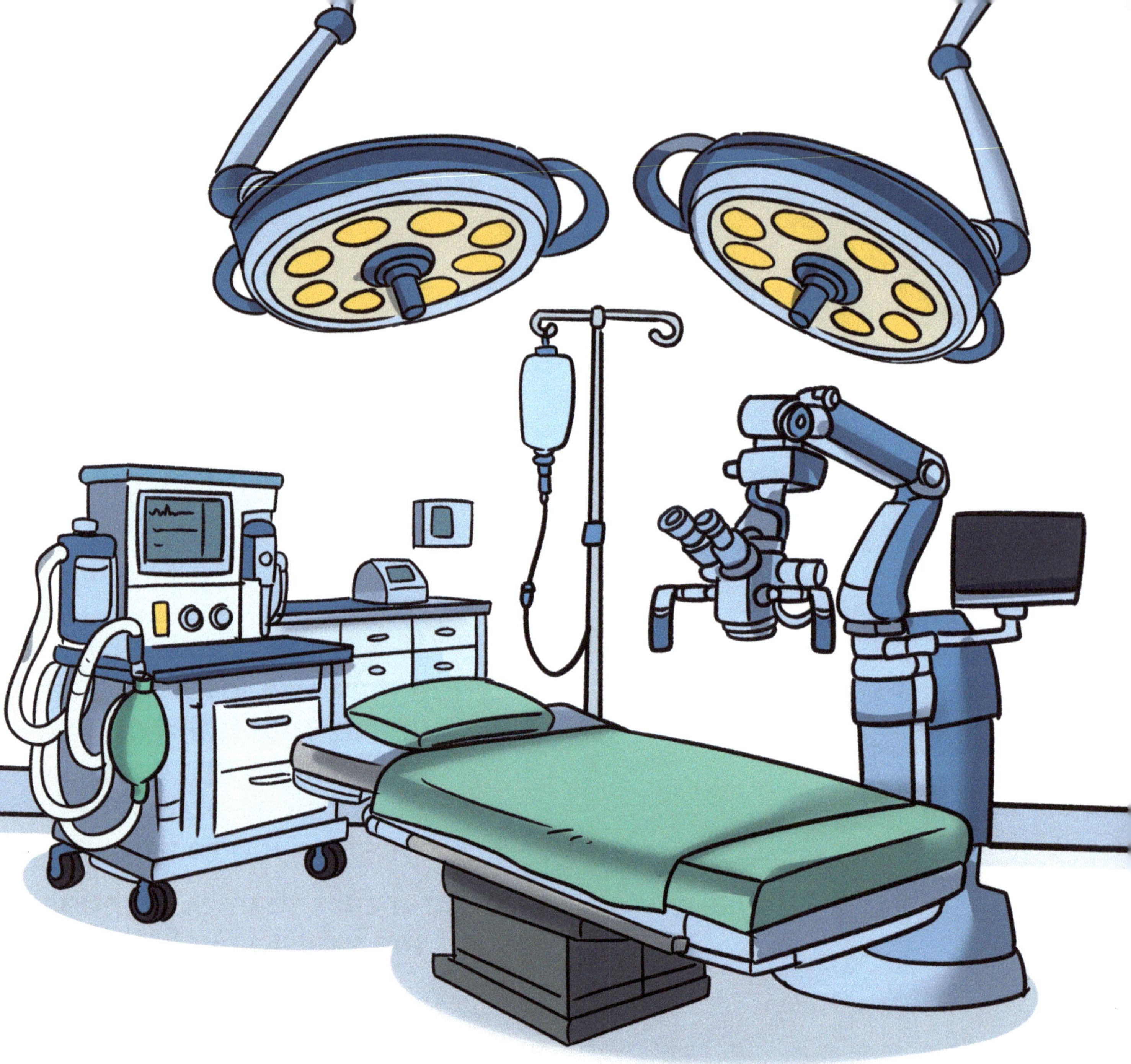

Let's check out the operating room
they have prepared just for you.

Can you spot these items in your room?

- [ ] The operating bed
- [ ] The anesthesia machine
- [ ] Big ceiling lights
- [ ] An IV pole
- [ ] A microscope (your doctor uses during brain surgery)
- [ ] Boxes of gloves
- [ ] A clock on the wall
- [ ] Different colored trash cans

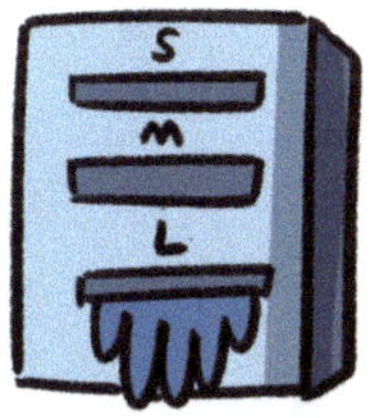

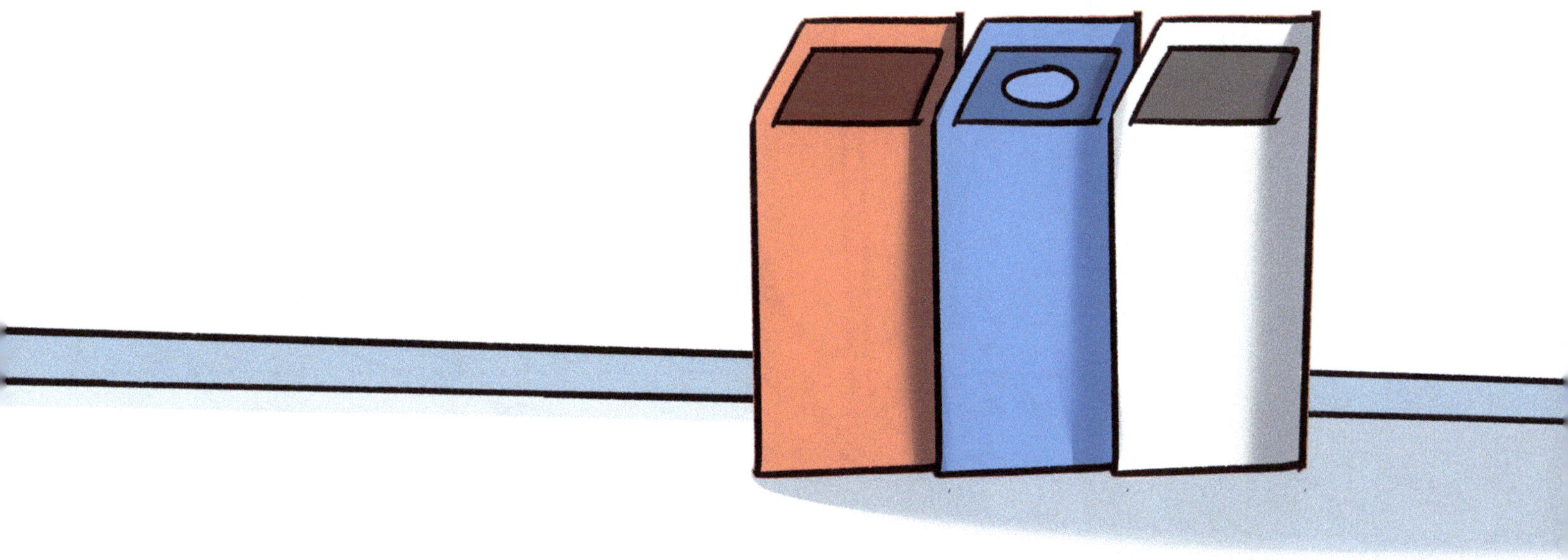

You can do this!

Some kids get the sleepy medicine through their IV.

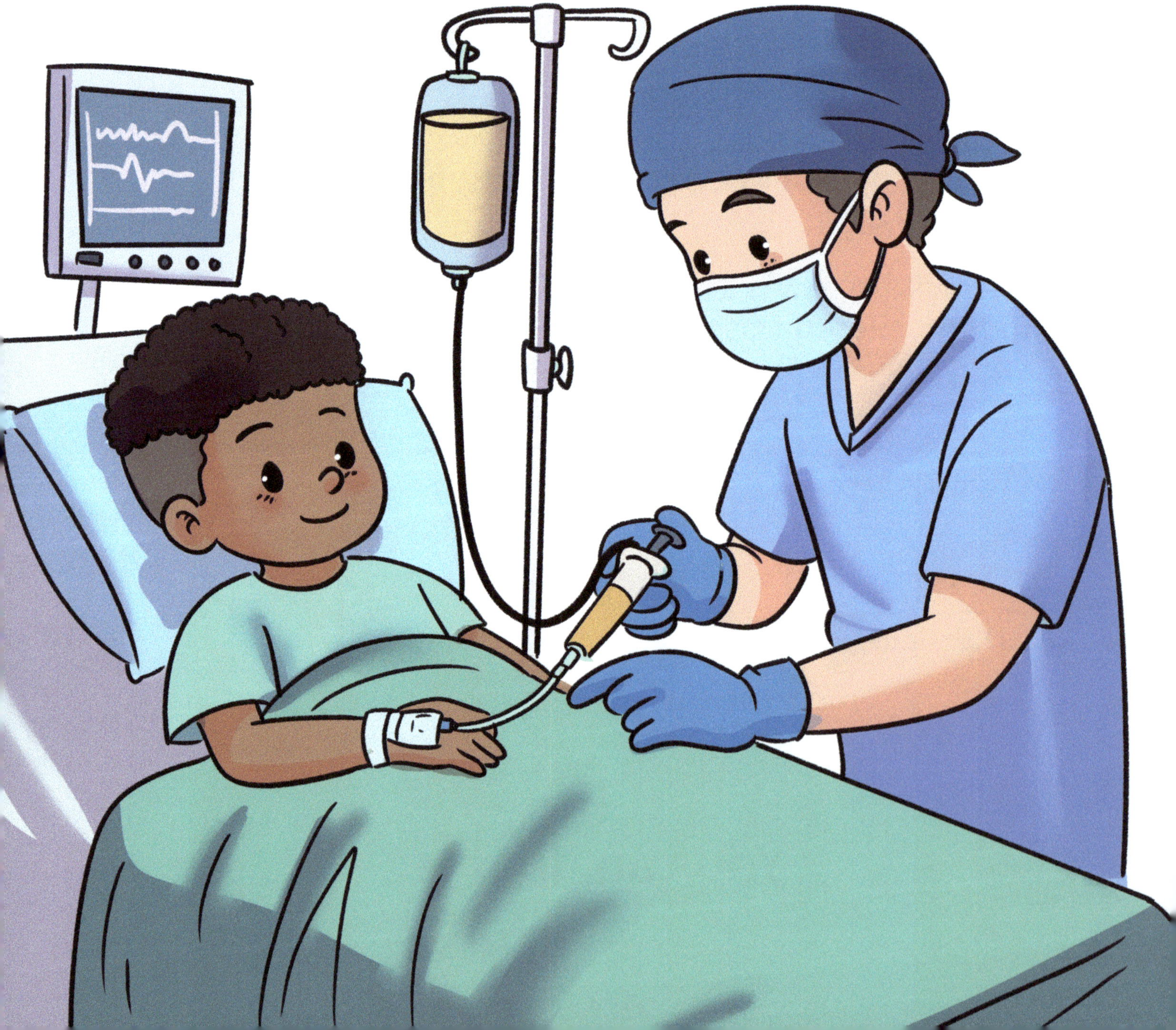

Some kids breathe it through a soft mask.

Your doctors and nurses will choose the safest way for you.

The medicine helps your body:

- Sleep deeply
- Feel no pain
- Stay very still.

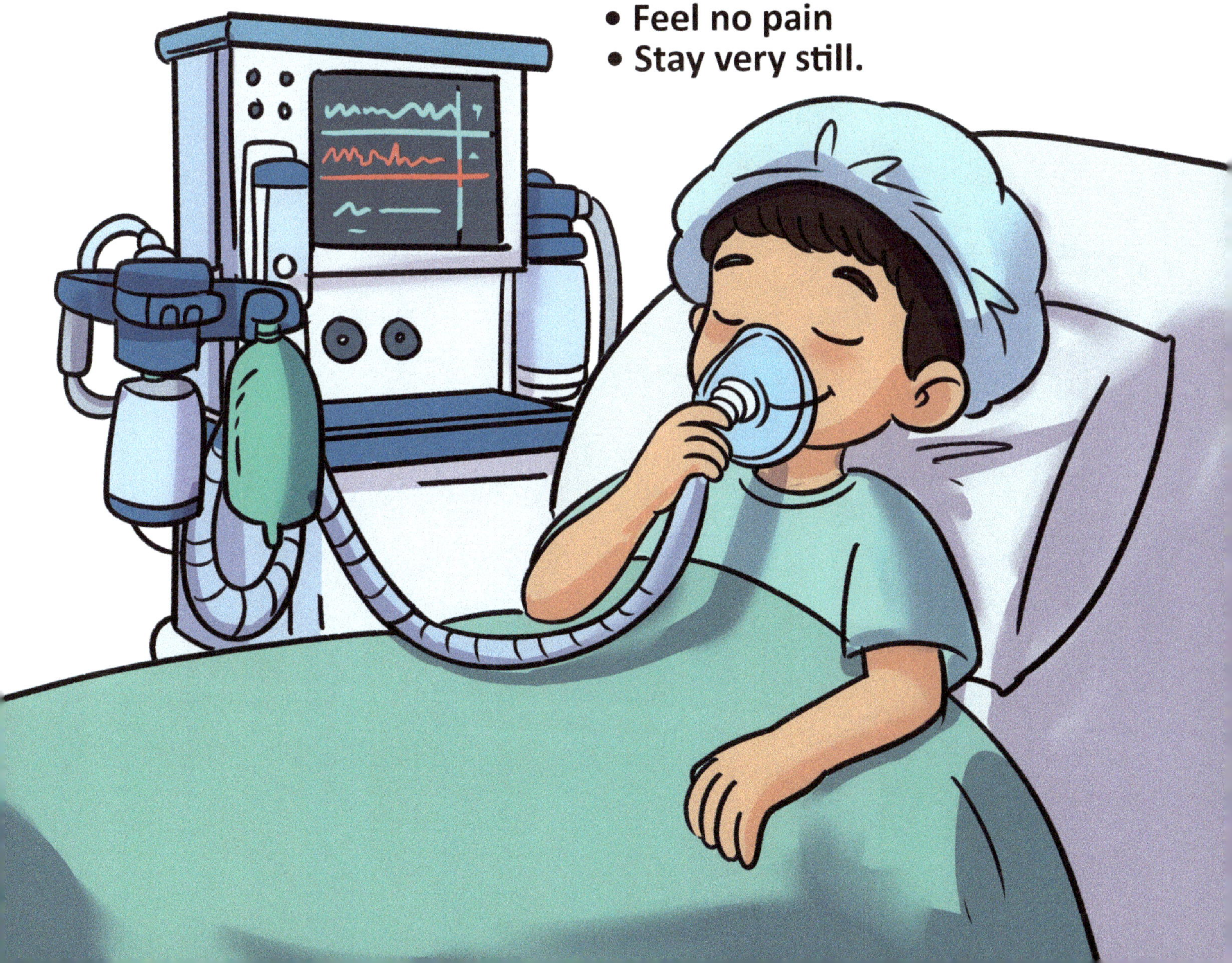

While you sleep, your doctor works gently and carefully.

Your surgery happens while you are sleeping,
and you won't feel a thing!

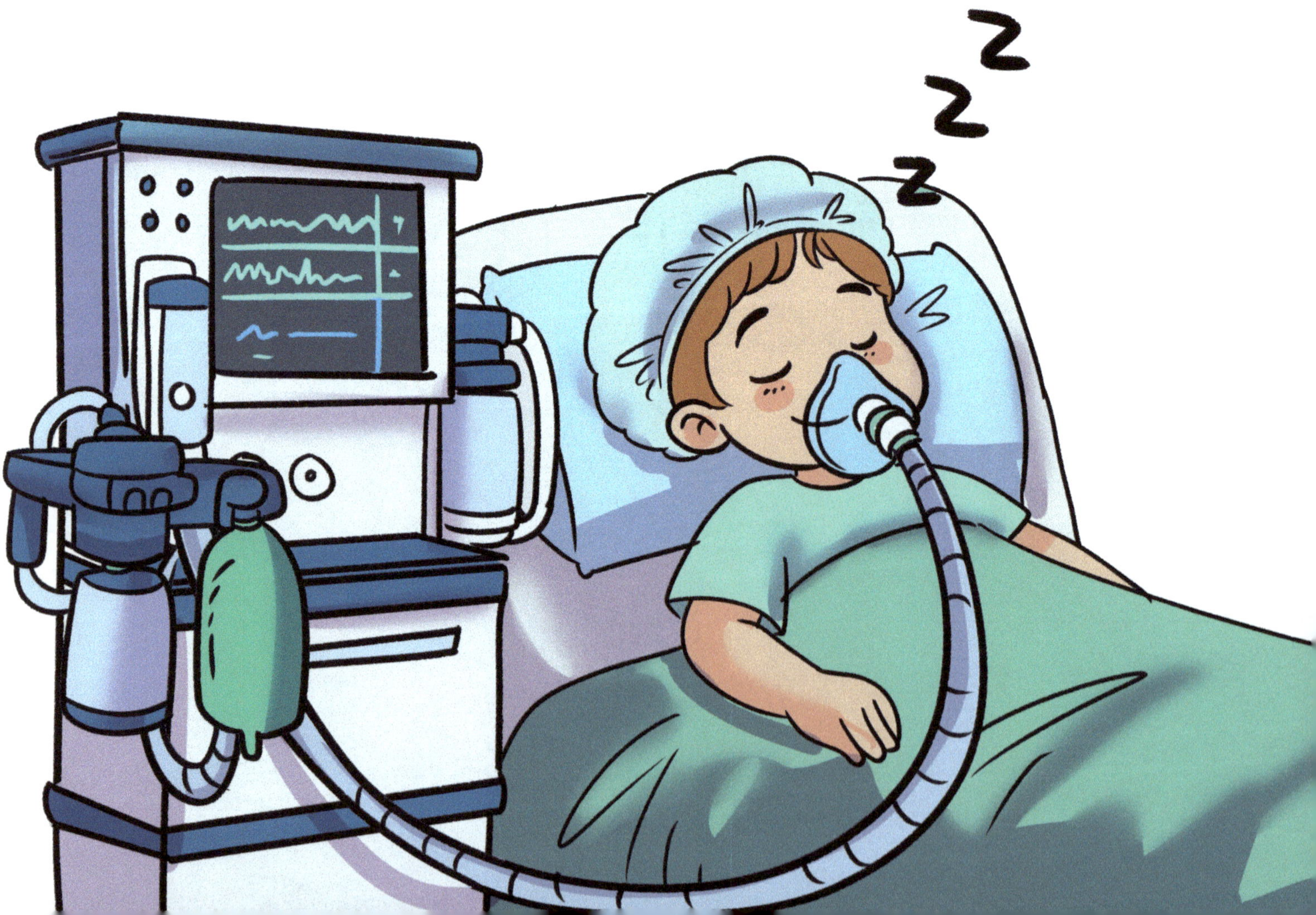

Your doctors and nurses will watch over you the whole time and keep you safe and comfortable.

What would you like to dream about?

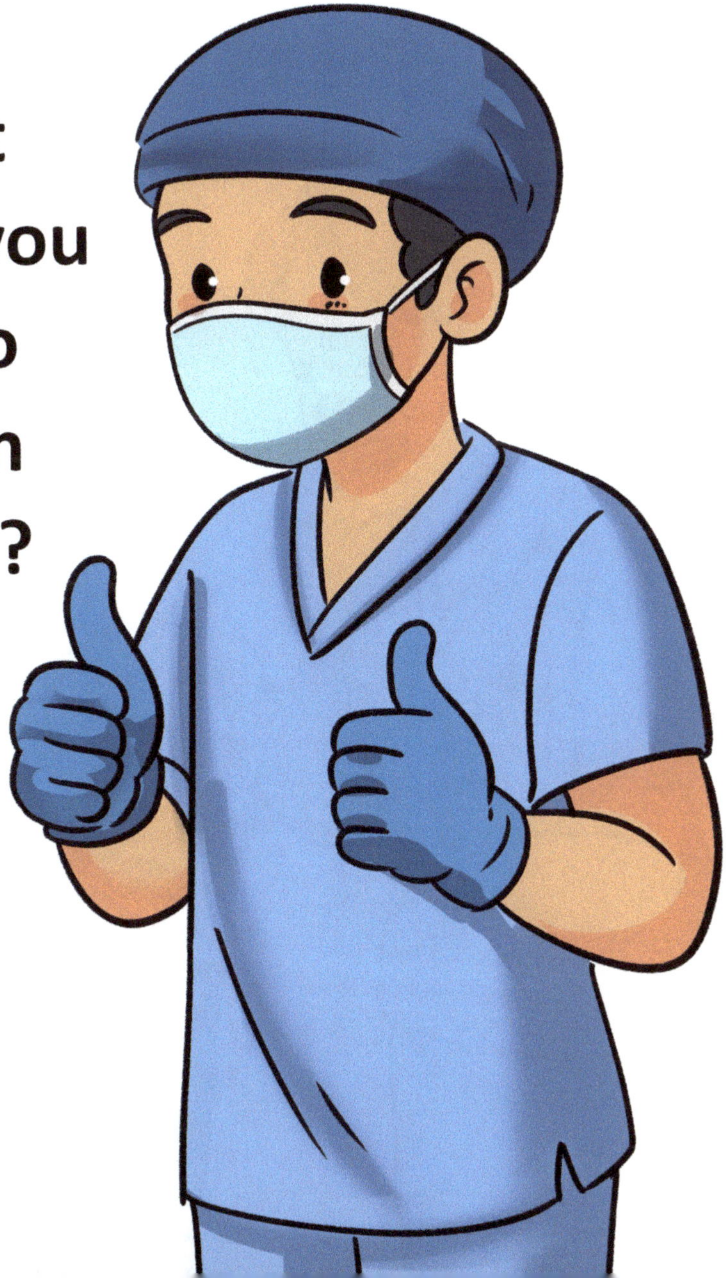

When you wake up, the surgery is already done.

You may hear beeping sounds.
They are just machines checking on you.

Your grown-up will be nearby.

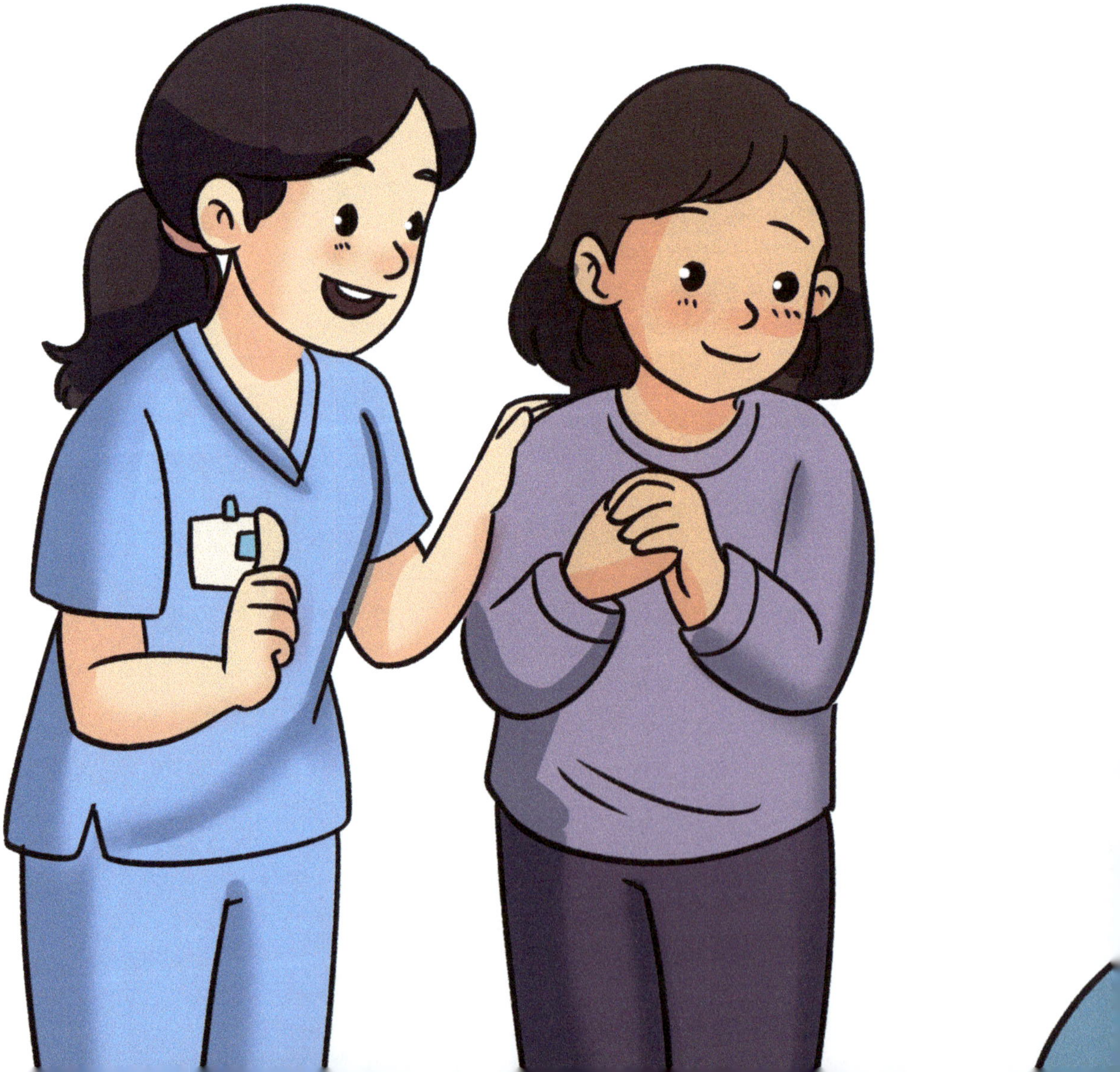

You may notice bandages or small tubes.
These are normal and help you heal.

You are so brave!

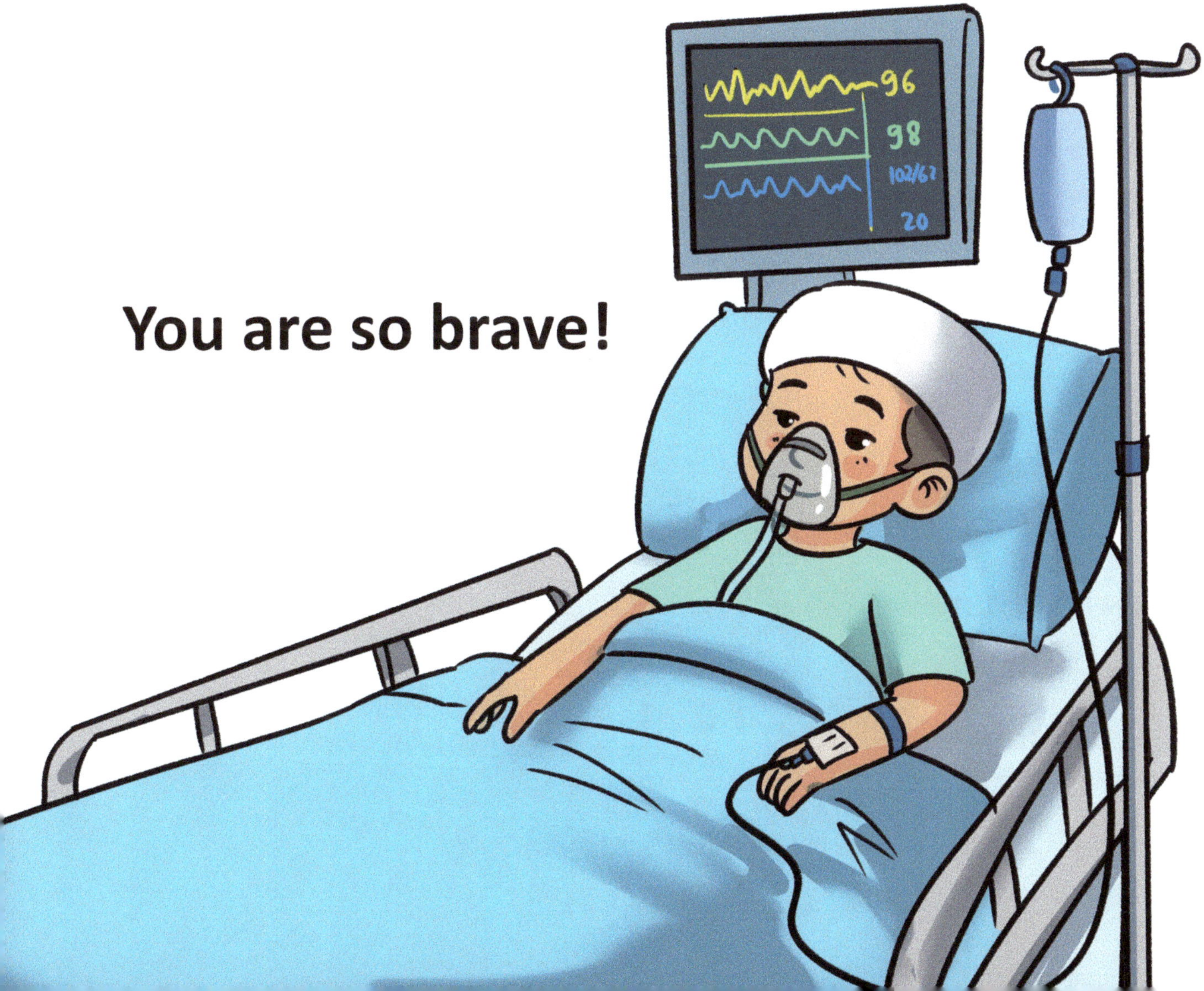

After surgery, you may:

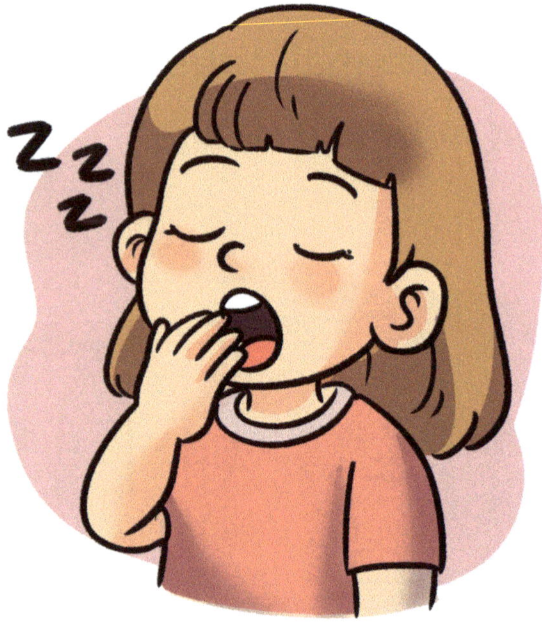

- Feel sleepy or tired

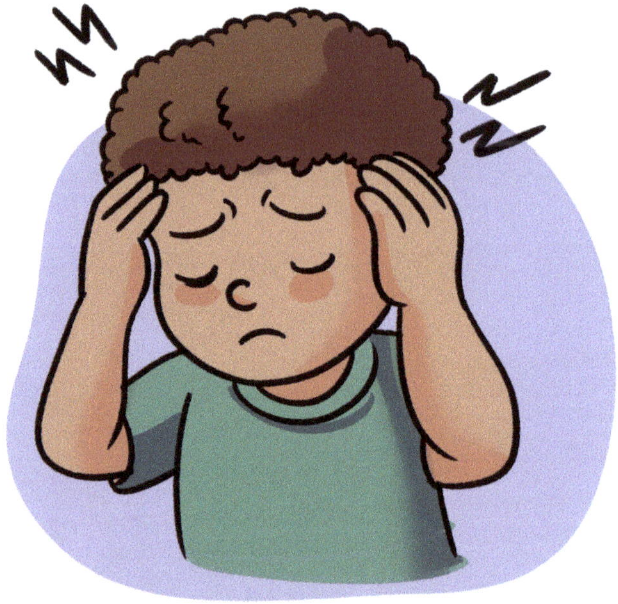

- Have a sore head or a headache

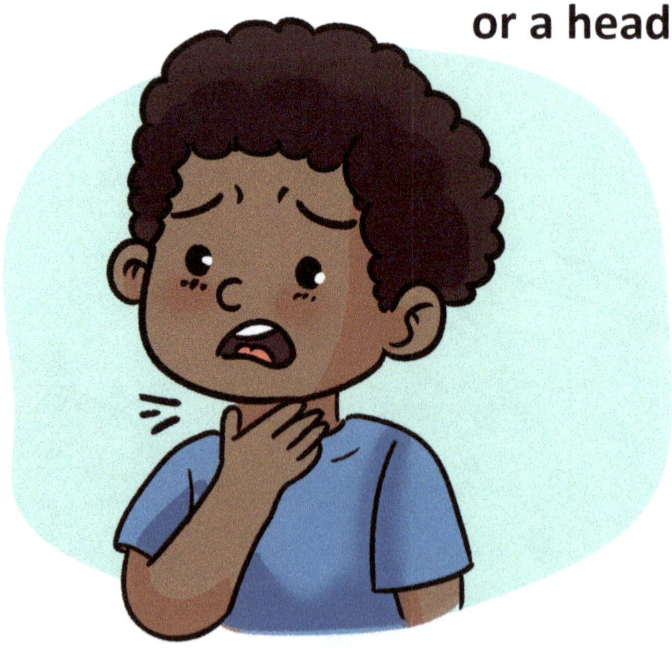

- Have a sore throat or feel sick to your tummy

- Feel dizzy or confused for a little while

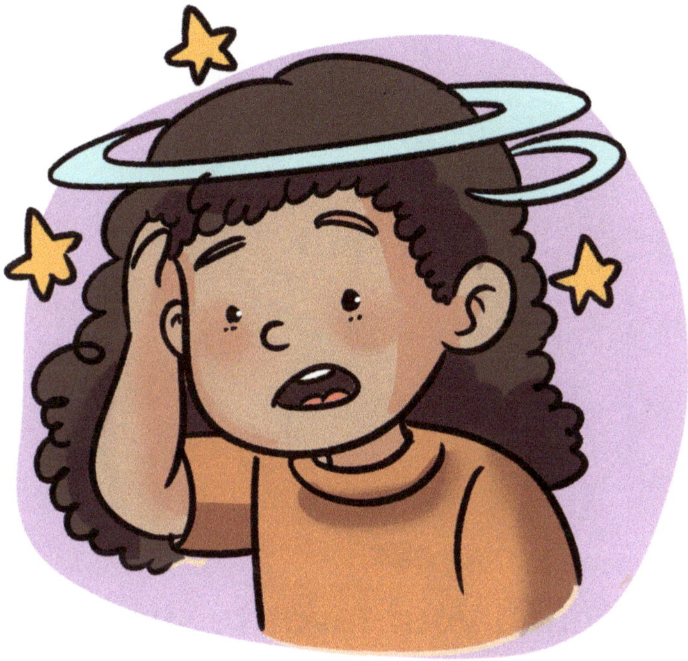

- Notice that some hair was trimmed (it will grow back)

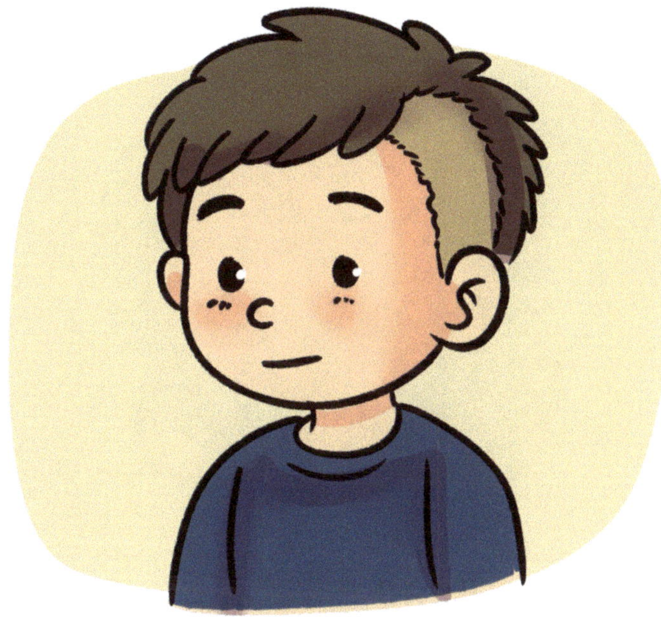

These feelings are normal.

Your body is healing, and it takes time.

Doctors and nurses will:
- Give you medicine to help with pain
- Check on you often
- Help you feel better

You may stay in the hospital for a few days until you're stronger and feeling better.

What helps you feel better?
Place a checkmark (✓) next to your favorites.

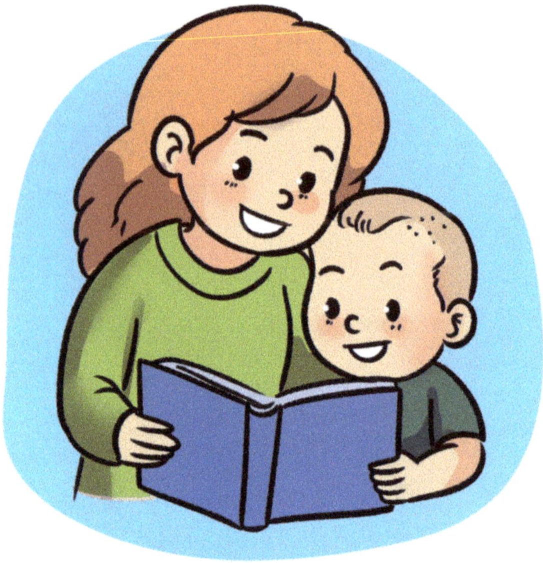

☐ Read a book

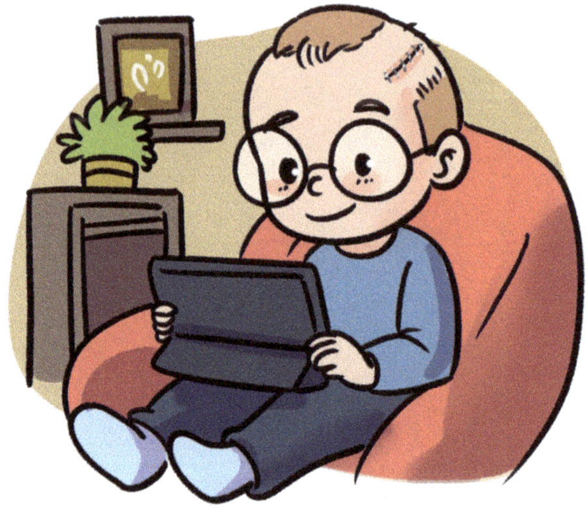

☐ Watch your favorite shows

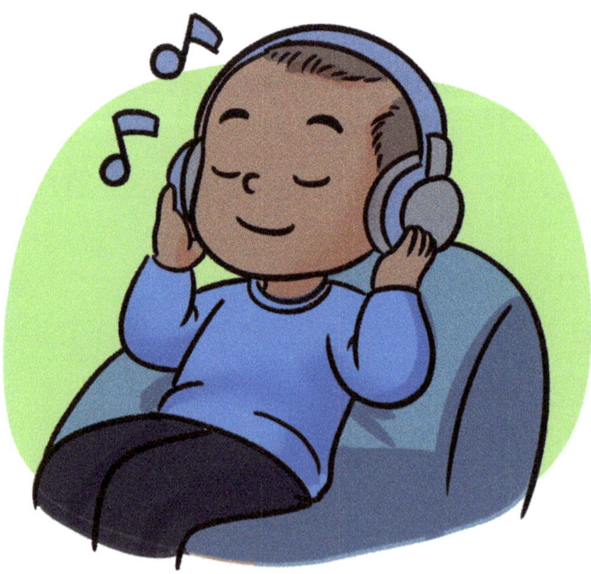

☐ Listen to your favorite songs

☐ Get a kiss or hug

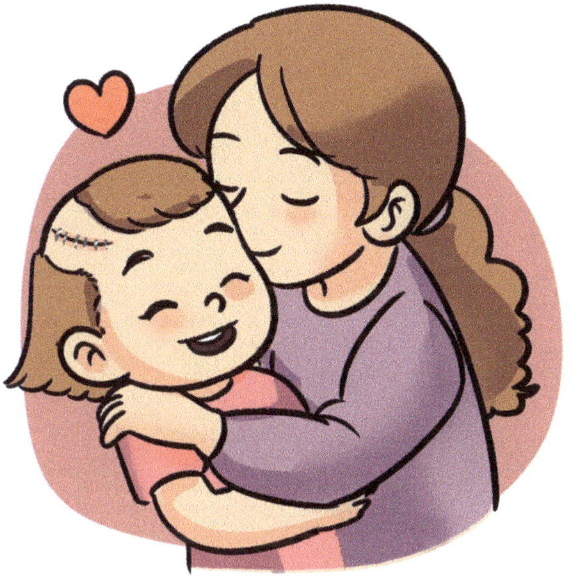

☐ Rest with your favorite blanket or stuffed animal

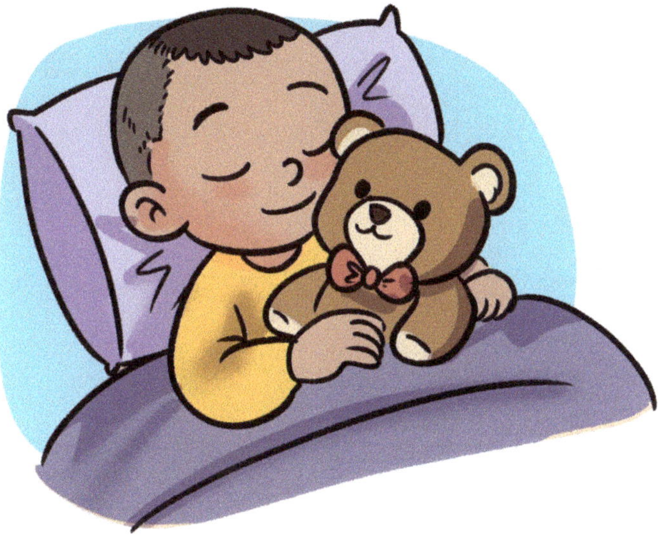

Take some medicine ☐

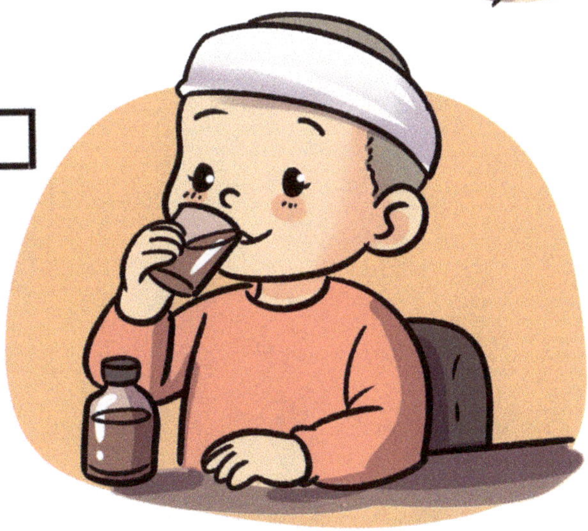

What creative ideas do you have to help you feel better?

You’ll see your doctor again to make sure you’re healing well.

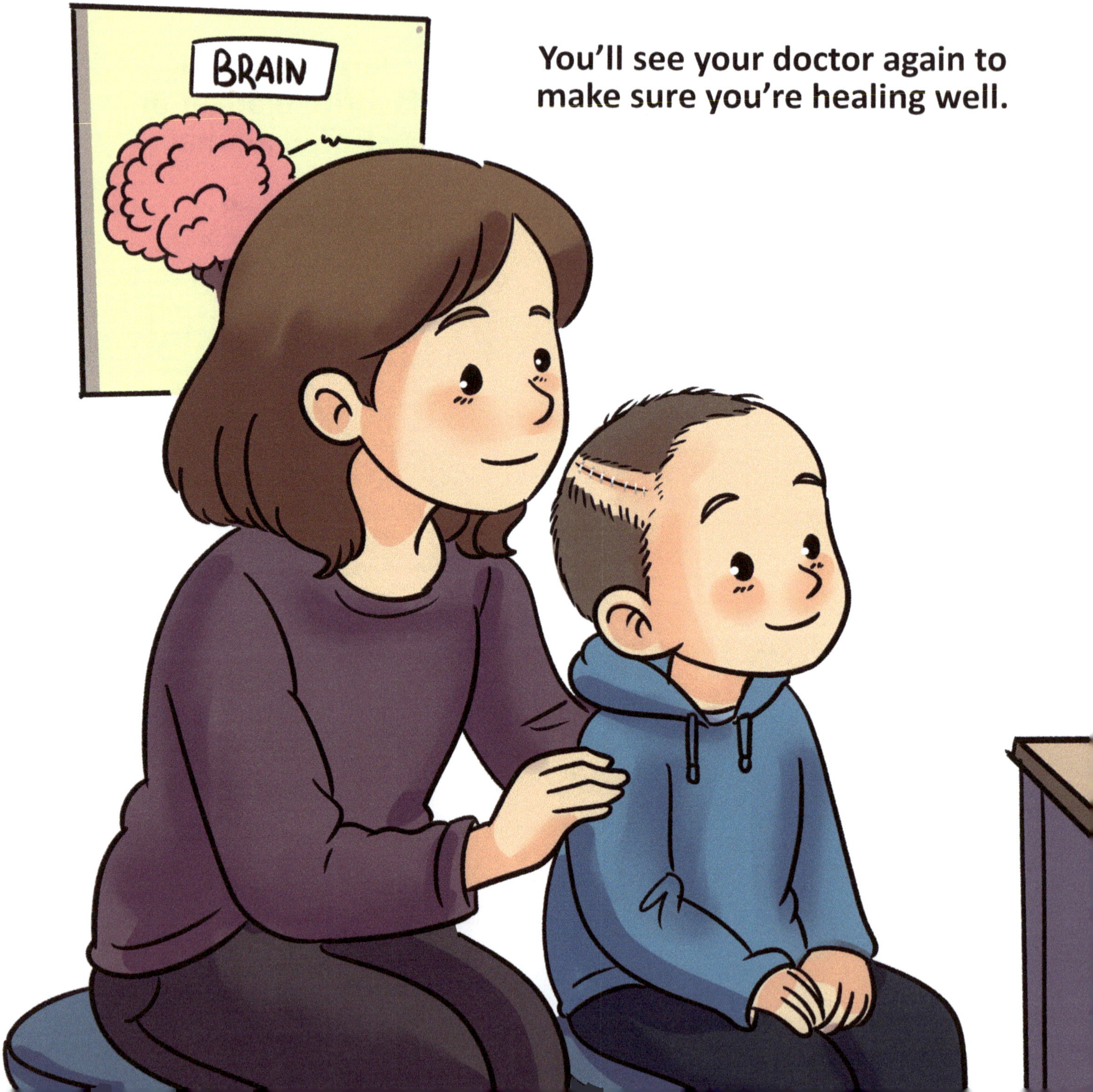

If you have questions, feel free to ask.

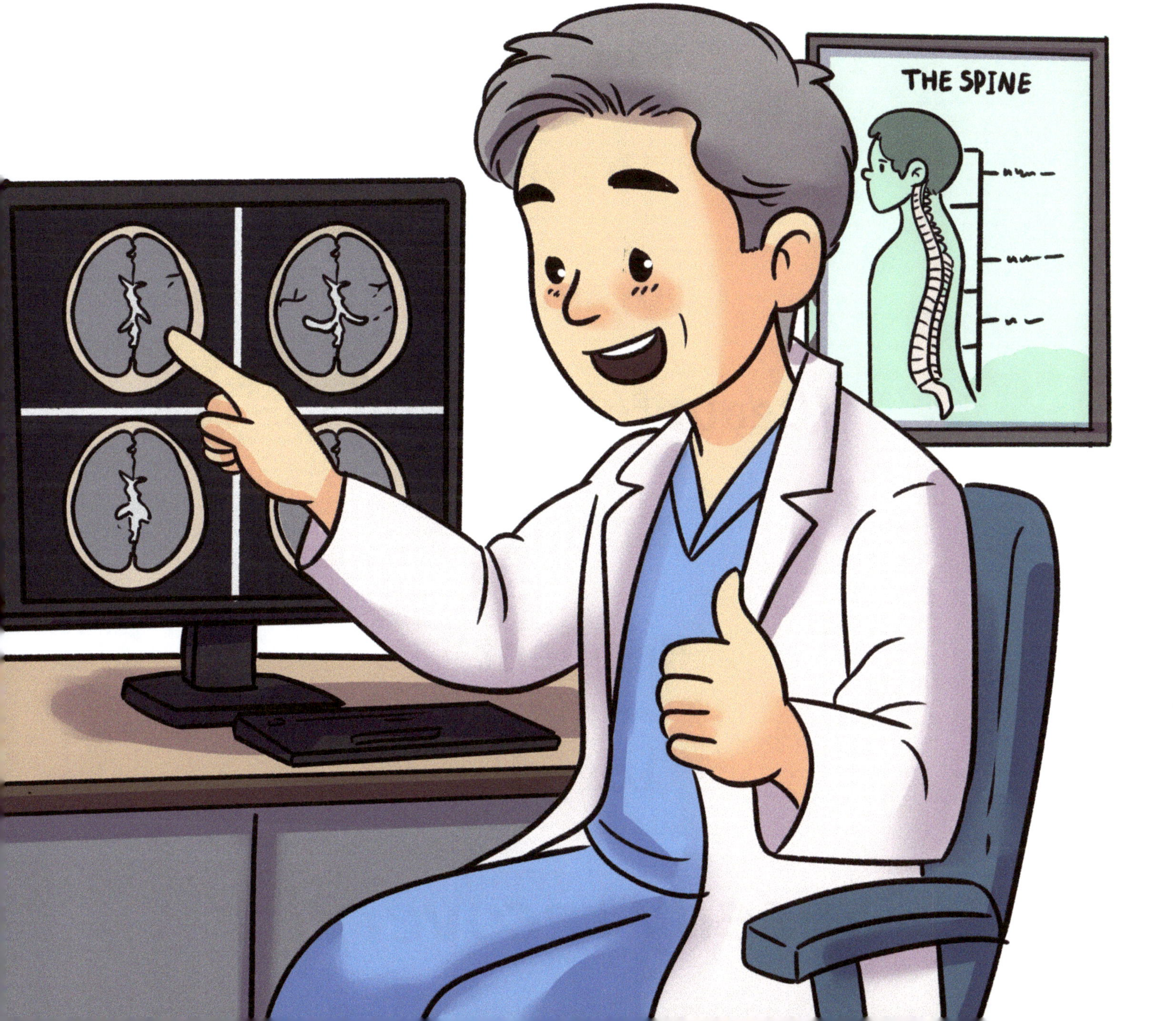

You are so brave.
Your brain is healing.
What's your favorite way to celebrate?

You are:

Brave

Courageous

Beautifully unique

Strong

Resilient

Loved

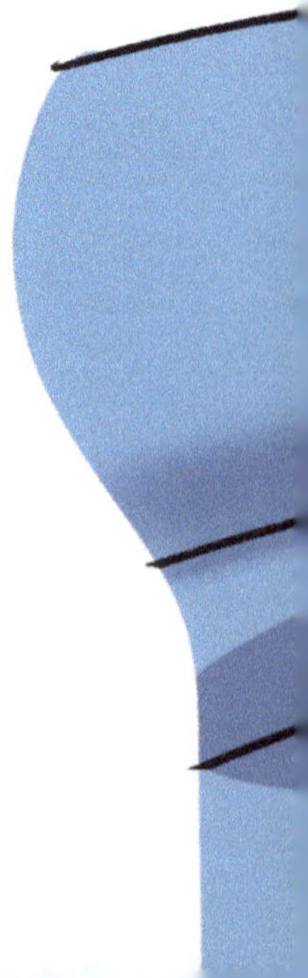

Speedy recovery!

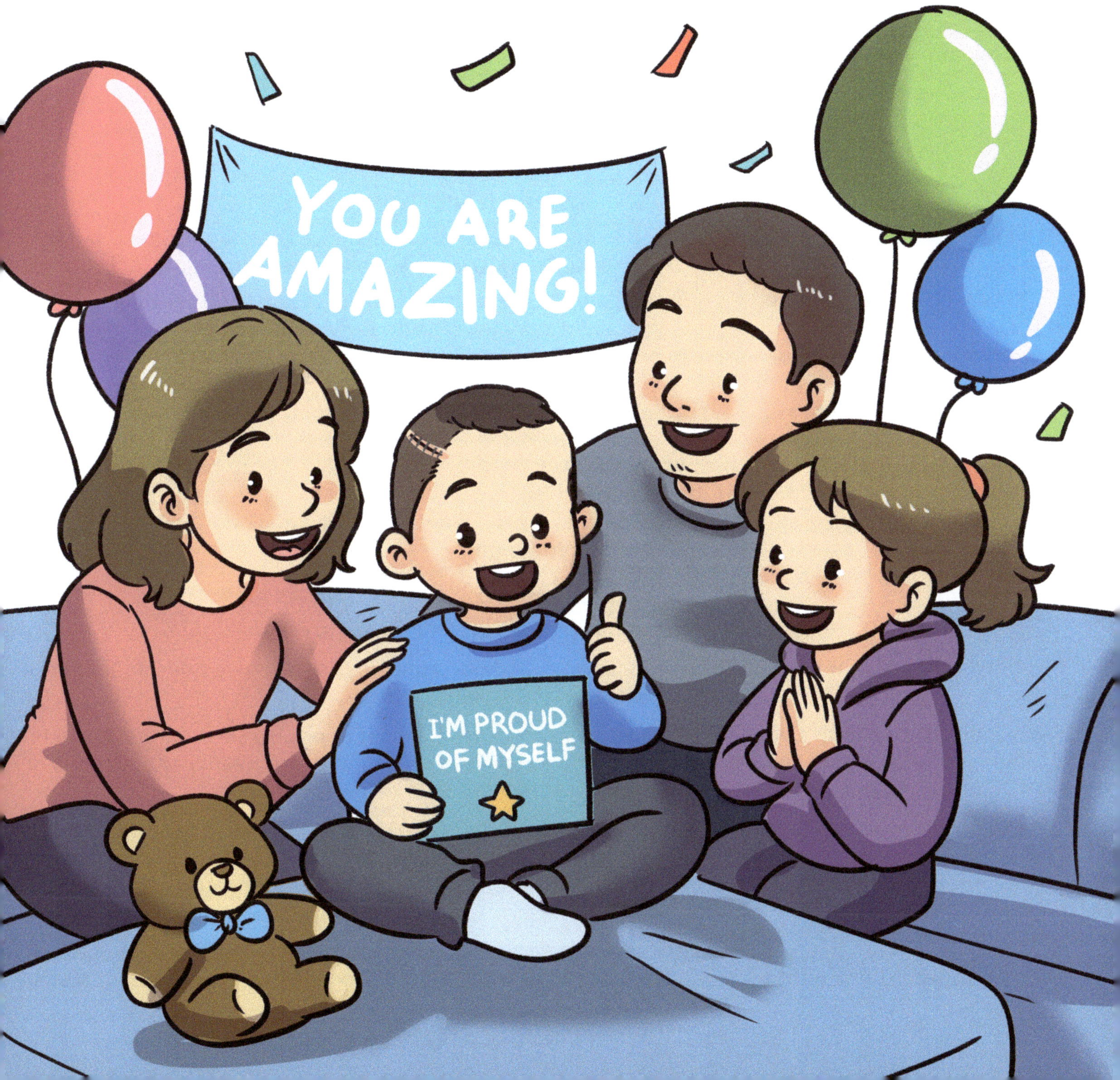
YOU ARE AMAZING!
I'M PROUD OF MYSELF

Notes for Parent/Guardian

Here is a list of foods and liquids and their corresponding times that need to pass between the time your child finishes eating or drinking them and the start of their surgery (from the American Society of Anesthesiologists):

Full meal or fatty foods: 8 hours
Infant formula or animal/plant milk: 6 hours
Breast milk: 4 hours
Clear liquids: 2 hours

Clear liquids are see-through liquids and some examples are apple juice (*not* apple cider), water, sugar water, and Pedialyte (*not* PediaSure). Orange juice is *not* a clear liquid.

Please note that every child is different, and it is important to discuss and confirm the above recommendations with your child's doctor prior to the day of surgery.

- If your child takes medicines regularly, please ask their doctor for instructions regarding the medicines for before and after the surgery.
- Placement of the intravenous (IV) catheter in this young age group is typically done *after* your child is asleep in the operating room with a face mask.
- Some children may stay in the hospital before surgery and may already have an IV in place. In these cases, anesthesia is often given through the IV instead of a face mask.
- Please do not shave your child's hair before surgery. If needed, this will be done safely in the operating room.

Disclaimer

Please note that the illustrations are not drawn to scale.

This book is written for informational, educational, and personal growth purposes and should not be used as a substitute for medical advice.

Please consult your child's doctor if they need medical attention and to ensure the information in this book pertains to your child's medical condition and needs. I cannot guarantee what your child experiences is exactly what is being discussed in this book.

The author and the publisher are not responsible, either directly or indirectly, for any damages, monetary losses, or reparations due to information in this book. By reading this book, the readers agree not to hold the author and the publisher responsible for any losses as a result of any errors, inaccuracies, or omissions in this book.

Please keep in mind that your child's experience depends on the location, the facility, their medical condition, and the healthcare team. Please use this book in conjunction with your child's doctor's advice. Thank you.

Did this picture book help your child in some way?
If so, I would love to hear about it!

www.amazon.com/gp/product-review/B0GZSYWRLW

For other book titles, please visit:

www.fzwbooks.com

Connect with the Author

email: books@fzwbooks.com
facebook/instagram: @FZWbooks

Books by the author

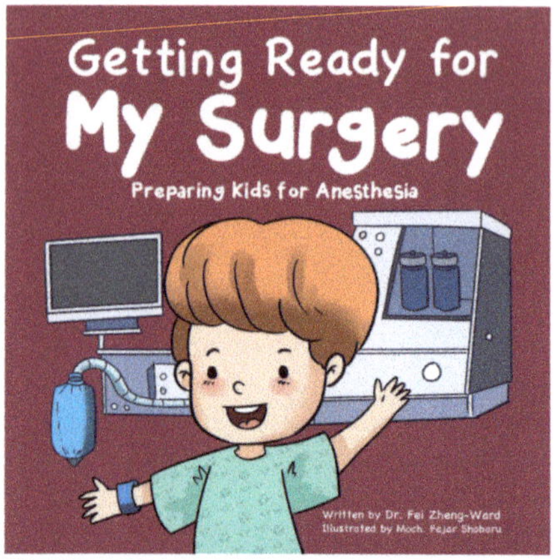

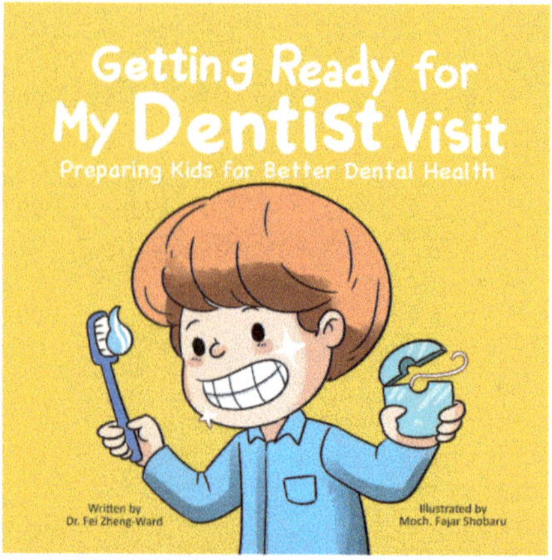

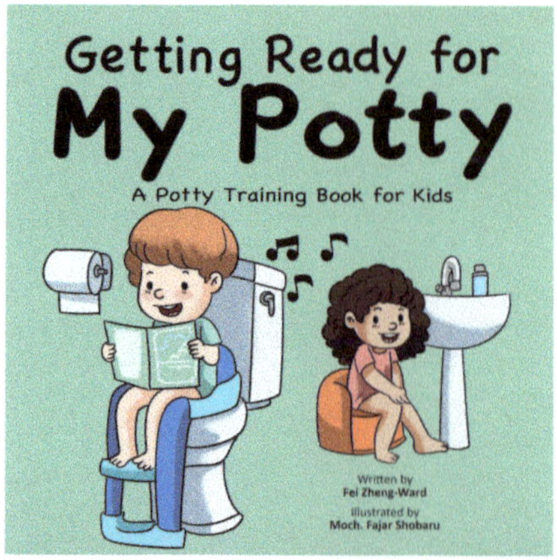

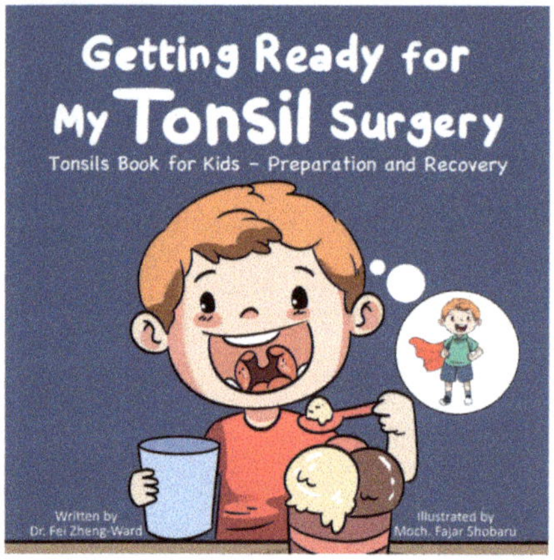

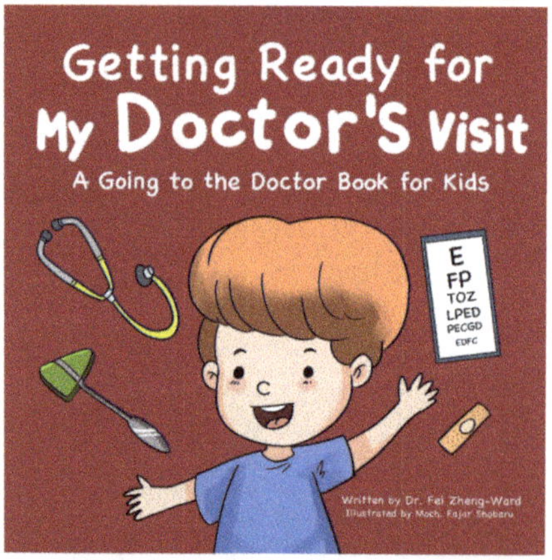

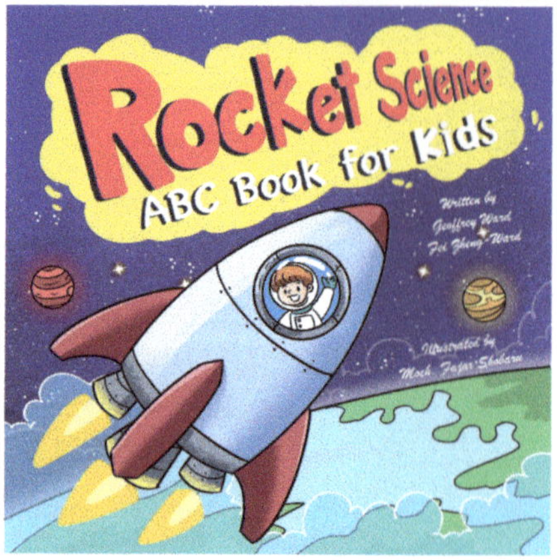

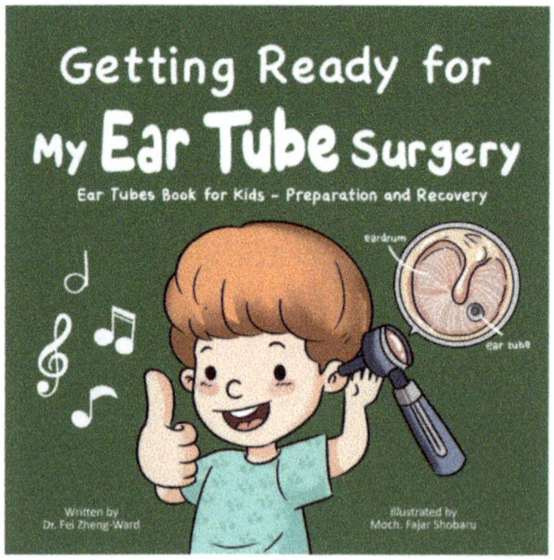

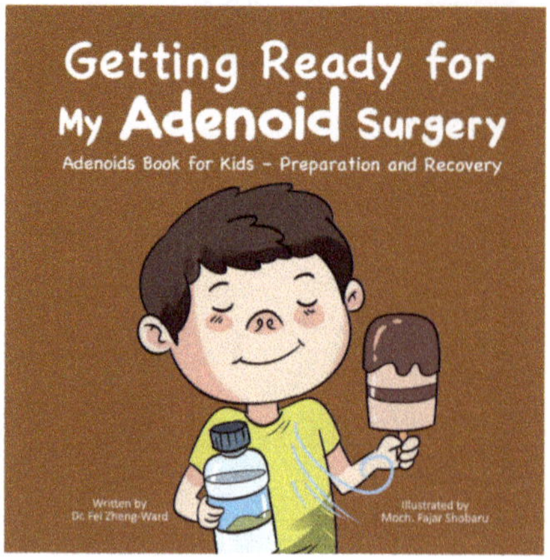

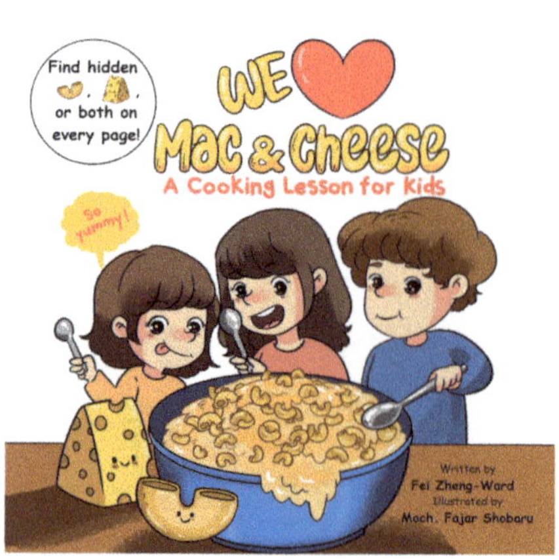

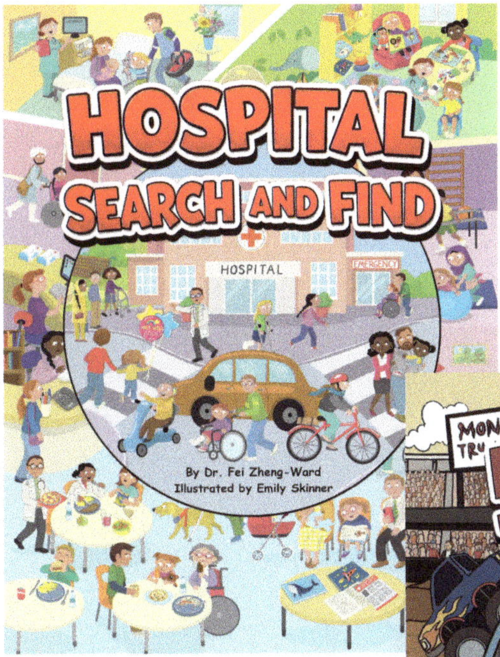
HOSPITAL
SEARCH AND FIND
HOSPITAL
EMERGENCY
By Dr. Fei Zheng-Ward
Illustrated by Emily Skinner

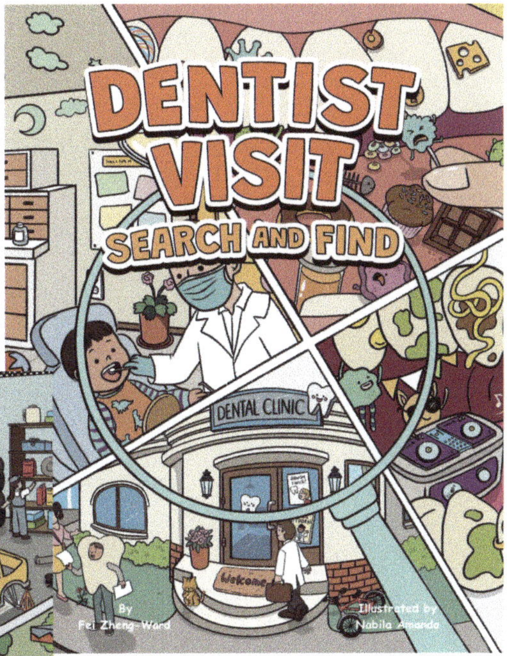
DENTIST
VISIT
SEARCH AND FIND
DENTAL CLINIC
Welcome
By
Fei Zheng-Ward
Illustrated by
Nabila Amanda

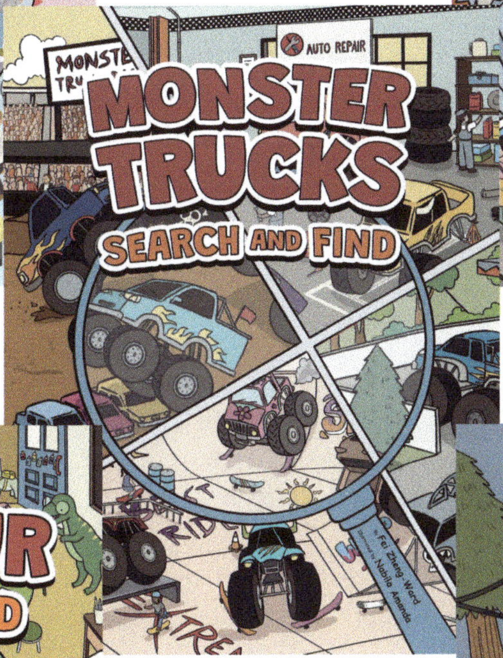
AUTO REPAIR
MONSTER
TRUCKS
SEARCH AND FIND

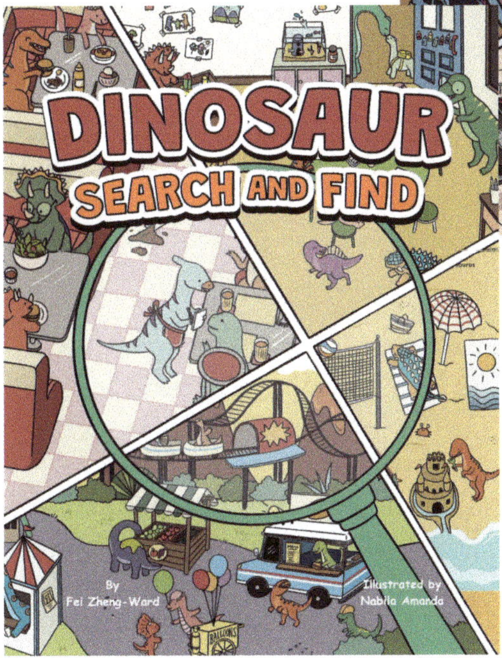
DINOSAUR
SEARCH AND FIND
By
Fei Zheng-Ward
Illustrated by
Nabila Amanda
BALLOONS

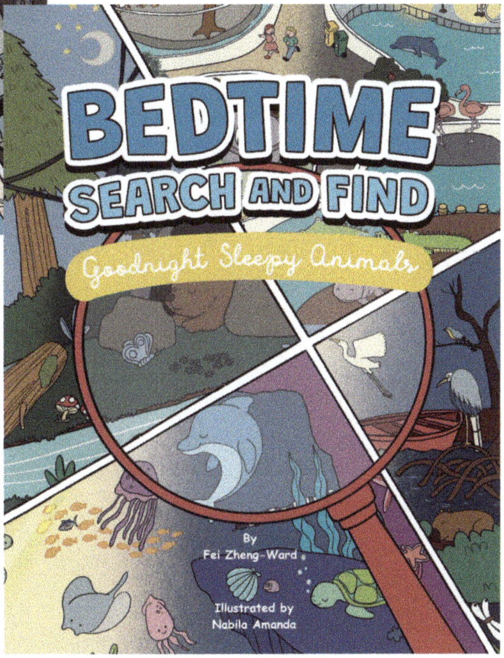
BEDTIME
SEARCH AND FIND
Goodnight Sleepy Animals
By
Fei Zheng-Ward
Illustrated by
Nabila Amanda

www.ingramcontent.com/pod-product-compliance
Lightning Source LLC
LaVergne TN
LVHW070911210926
848482LV00017B/1053
* 9 7 9 8 8 9 3 1 8 1 8 3 8 *